ARISE Basic Health 101: Nutrition and Exercise

Instructor's Manual

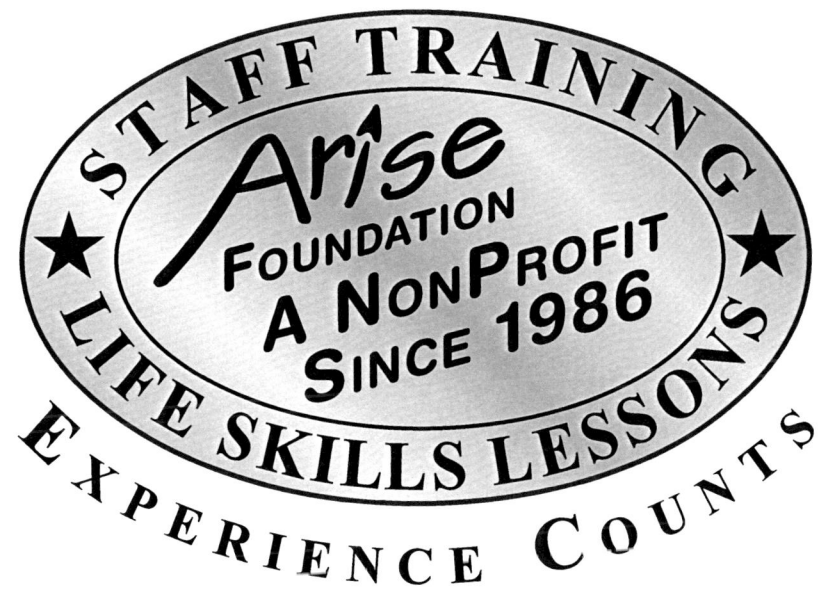

ariselife-skills.org

COPYRIGHT

Without limiting the rights under copyright reserved above, no part of this publication may be reproduced, stored in, or introduced into a retrieval system, or transmitted, in any form or by any means (electronic, mechanical, photocopying, recording, or otherwise) without the prior written permission of both the copyright owner and the above publisher of this book. © 1996-2011-2014 ARISE Foundation. All Rights Reserved.

ARISE Foundation makes no representation or warranties of any kind, either expressed or implied, including, but not limited to, the warranties of fitness for a particular purpose and/or merchantability for services provided. ARISE Foundation is not responsible for any damages suffered from the use of its services or materials under any circumstances whatsoever.

> Special imprints, messages, and excerpts can be produced to meet your needs. For more information, contact us.

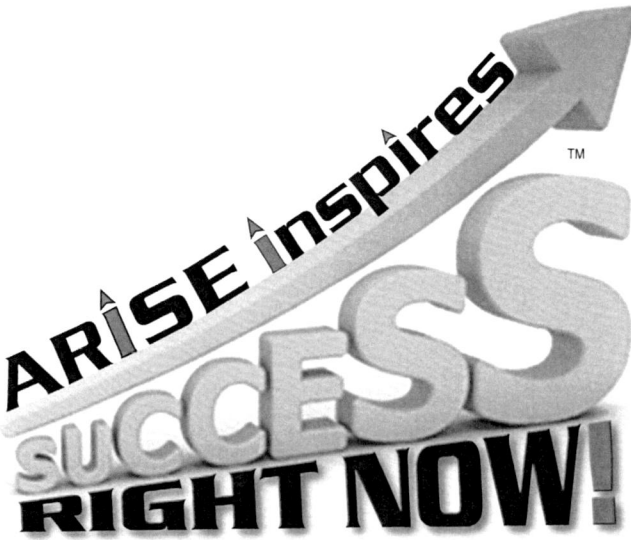

ariselife-skills.org   ARISE Adds Value to Lives   Toll-Free: 1-888-680-6100

ARISE Basic Health 101: Nutrition and Exercise
Table of Contents

ARISE Foundation: An Overview..3
What Are People Saying About ARISE?..4
Tips for Teaching ARISE Life Management Skills..6
Performance Evaluation...7

SECTION ONE
Introduction..10
Eating Well...11
Food Facts..13
Eating Disorders...15
Review Activity..17

SECTION TWO
Introduction..18
MyPlace..19
Nutrients I..21
Nutrients II..23
Review Activity..25

SECTION THREE
Introduction..26
Being Physically Fit...27
Exercise..29
Flexibility and Strength...31
Review Activity..33
Worth Remembering..34

NOTE TO INSTRUCTORS
PLEASE COPY THE VOCABULARY LIST ON PAGES **98** AND **99** FOR THE LEARNERS IF YOU DO NOT HAVE THE COMPANION LEARNER'S WORKBOOK. OTHERWISE, THE VOCABULARY LIST CAN BE FOUND ON PAGES **67** AND **68** OF THE LEARNER'S WORKBOOK.

ARISE Basic Health 101: Nutrition and Exercise

Table of Contents (cont.)

Learner's Worksheets

SECTION 1	37
SECTION 2	59
SECTION 3	79
Vocabulary	98

Quizzes, Assessments, Answer Keys and Bonus Material

Worksheet Answers	100
Quizzes and Assessments	106
Quiz and Assessment Answers	112
Discussion Questions and Activity Ideas for the ARISE Inspirational Biographies	115
ARISE Inspirational Biographies	116
Vision Board Activity	119
Using ARISE True Life Tales to Create Memorable Learning Experiences	120
ARISE True Life Tales	121
Mind Map Activity	129
Comic Activity	130
How to Make the Most of the ARISE Life Quotes Found Throughout This Manual	131
How to Effectively Use the ARISE Motivational Posters in This Manual	132
ARISE Motivational Posters	133
ARISE Curricula and Training	137

ARISE Foundation: An Overview

Our Mission
- Providing young men and women with the tools they need to survive, succeed, and become super-productive members of society.
- Educating and motivating young adults by equipping them with practical information they can use every single day of their lives.
- Helping youth achieve their highest potential by enriching their own lives and those they interact with.

History of Success
For more than 25 years, ARISE has operated as a developer and publisher of life-skills curricula and staff training programs. Designed originally to reach at-risk incarcerated youth in detention centers and secure facilities, ARISE is also used as a powerful prevention tool for teenagers and young adults. ARISE is particularly appropriate for youth with special requirements and limited reading and/or writing ability. It has been successfully used for over 25 years in the Miami-Dade school system and in over 100 Washington, D.C. schools, organizations, and secure facilities. ARISE is also being used across the United States, in Canada, Jamaica, England, Australia, Bahamas, Bermuda, New Zealand, Mexico, Puerto Rico, Bosnia, Kazakhstan, Kingdom of Bahrain, and Central Asia and more.

To date, ARISE has trained over 5,000 Certified Life-Skills Instructors, who have taught more than 4,800,000 hours of interactive, boredom-busting, and statistically proven lessons to over hundreds of thousands of high-risk youth.

What's Different about ARISE?
- Lessons are fun and interactive, never boring. No one sits quietly on the sidelines because the learners are involved in activities. They learn from each other, with activities that are engaging, such as role-playing, brainstorming, and group discussions.
- Perfect for those with reading difficulties. All workbook pages are easy to read, but the intellectual level of discussion is much higher.
- Each lesson is self-contained and not dependent on previously learned material. The students do not have to know anything about the subject when they enter your class.
- Start anywhere in ARISE; learners are able to jump into the action on their first day in class.
- Material can be used during school, after school, and on weekends…use it every day.
- ARISE curricula available as print or e-book.

WHAT ARE PEOPLE SAYING ABOUT ARISE?

Yashtina, Learner, Dade Regional Juvenile Detention Center, Miami, FL

"I enjoy working in these books because they're fun and easy to do. Everything I'm going through is in these books."

Anthony, Learner, Palm Beach Juvenile Correctional Facility, West Palm Beach, FL

"ARISE taught me how to pick friends who I can trust. I learned that my past mistakes can hurt other people and that my past mistakes are in the past. I learned that I could change while I am here and that I can succeed in life and in my community. I also learned that I have to make better choices in life. I also learned that I have to have empathy for others and to be accountable for my mistakes."

Flora Johnson, Teacher, Dade Marine Institute South, Miami, FL

"The training was very educational, informative and interesting."

Raymond Mincey, Officer, Metro Police, District of Columbia

"I found the information on how to get students more involved with the instructional activities and keeping their attention during the class most helpful. I enjoyed the training and look forward to the chance of sharing the ARISE methods of learning with my students."

The following guideline gives you an idea of how long it should take to complete this ARISE book:

> An ARISE-trained instructor would be able to teach approximately 36 group sessions (or more) with each book, assuming group sessions last 45 minutes to an hour. This means that if ARISE groups are taught three times per week, a book should last a minimum of 12 weeks. If ARISE groups are taught five times per week, a single book should last 7 weeks.

Guidelines for a group session:

BEFORE ARISE GROUP SESSION

Things to do and say as your group session begins:
- Explain how the group will operate. Stress that this program is interactive. Learners will be expected to participate fully through brainstorming, role-playing, discussion, and other activities.

DURING ARISE GROUP SESSION

- Have learners form small groups of three or four for most activities. Remember to mix them up; don't always place the same people together. For other exercises, they will be in pairs. Pair the more active learners with the less responsive ones.
- Do the worksheets together by reading the questions out loud. They will brainstorm to come up with answers.
- With quizzes, make sure the instructions you give are clear and complete. Read the quiz questions to everyone.

AFTER ARISE GROUP SESSION

As you reach the end of the group session, do the following:
- Write the *Worth Remembering* thoughts (found on pages 34 and 35 of this manual) on the board or on a large piece of paper. Read the quotes out loud, *twice*, to all. Ask them to think about the meaning. Discuss their opinions. Encourage everyone to talk about these ideas.
- Ask the group what they got out of the session each day. Encourage feedback. Find out what else they would like to learn about this subject.

TIPS FOR TEACHING ARISE LIFE MANAGEMENT SKILLS

You are about to undertake a real challenge: trying to change a human being's behavior and way of thinking. We refer to students as "learners" in our books. Over the years, we have found the following tips very helpful in teaching ARISE Life Management Skills:

1. Be energetic. The livelier and more enthusiastic you are, the more involved learners will be.

2. Pay attention to learners' reading levels. Match your language to them and avoid commenting on their spelling or grammar.

3. Be positive. Make certain that the learners' experience with you and this program is one of success. Praise them at every possible turn, even if their responses are inappropriate. Say things like:

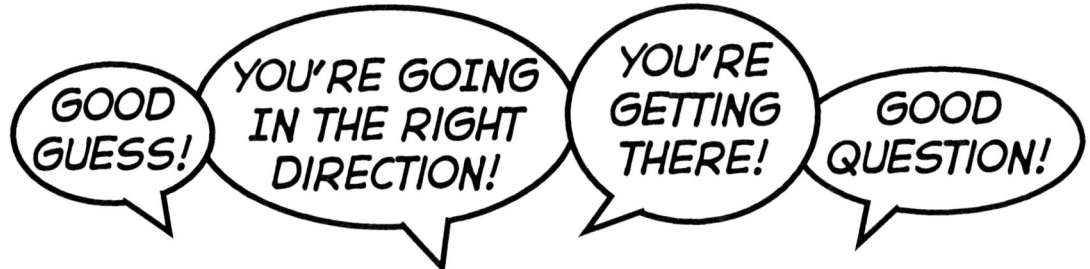

4. Every opinion is valuable and any answer, no matter how off the wall, demonstrates the individual is paying attention. So praise *all* efforts. The objective of ARISE Life Management Skills is for everyone to participate and absorb the material.

5. Be kind. *Never* lecture to learners. Rather, *explain* to them. Talk with the group. Listen patiently.

6. Make yours an active class. Move around from time to time. Encourage the group to take part in role-playing, dramatizing stories, developing skits and songs, and all other ARISE Life Management Lessons.

7. Research by industrial training professionals indicates that people retain information better when they hear it rather than read it; and when they hear *and* see it, the retention rate improves by 40%. And, when we stand up and read, the mind works even better. So, to put it all together, when you want to really recall something you are reading, *read out loud while standing up.*

PERFORMANCE EVALUATION

This program is not based on how well people learn the answers to quizzes. Rather, this program is considered successful when learners have participated fully and enthusiastically in class, when they have learned to think a little differently, and when they have enjoyed being part of the program.

In order to assess learners' participation, observe them during class. Record your observations as soon as possible while your recollections are fresh. Use a notepad to record what you observe.

Remember: Just asking the learners to create pictures and stories is not enough. Learners MUST be asked to volunteer to read or show off their work. Otherwise, they will think we are wasting their time. There must be an outlet for their creativity.

How to observe:
- Focus your observation on a few learners at a time.
- Observe learners at the beginning of the group session, while it is in progress, and at the end of the session.
- Observe learners when they are working as individuals, as a partner, or as part of a group.

What to observe:
- Observe which learners understand new concepts.
- Observe which learners need extra support.
- Observe which learners contribute to conversation or activity.
- Observe which learners interact and how they interact.

What you will gain through observation:
- How to identify learners' strengths.
- How to recognize areas that need improvement.
- How to set goals together in areas that need to be developed.
- How to provide needed feedback to learners themselves.

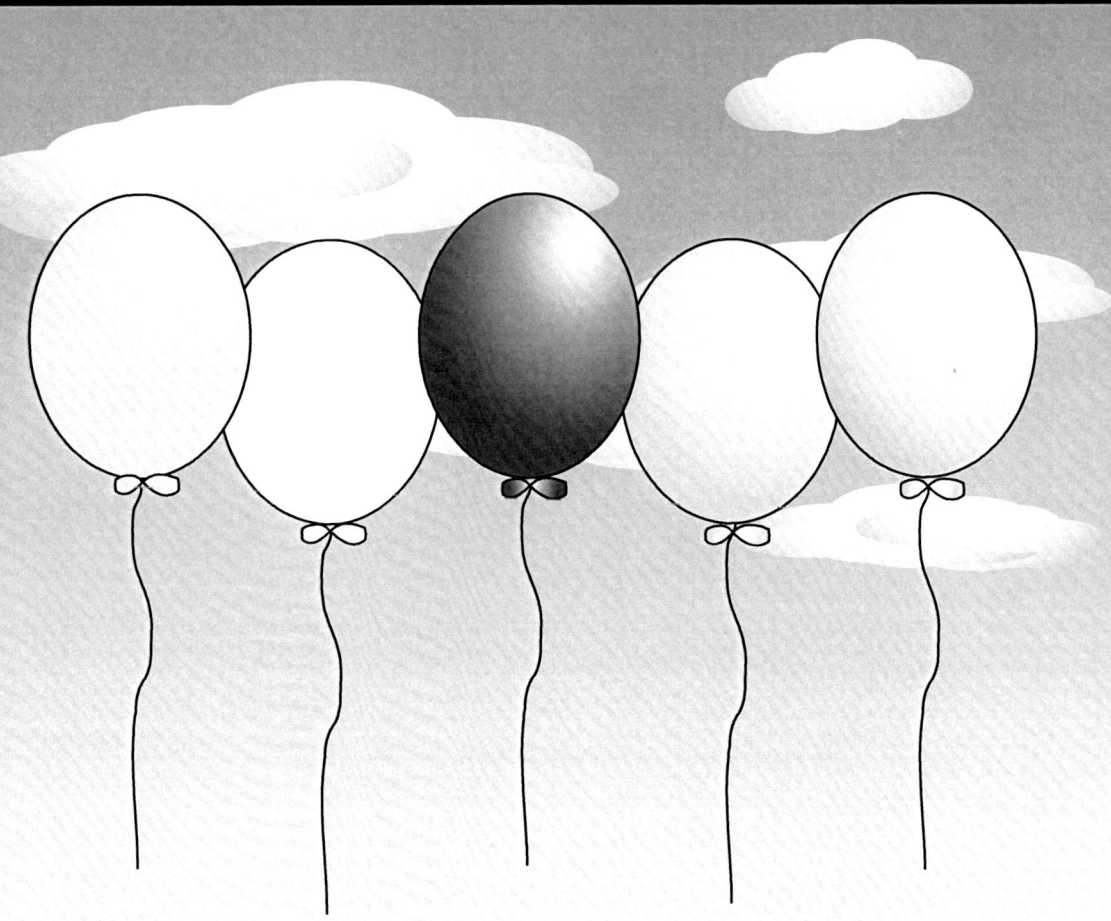

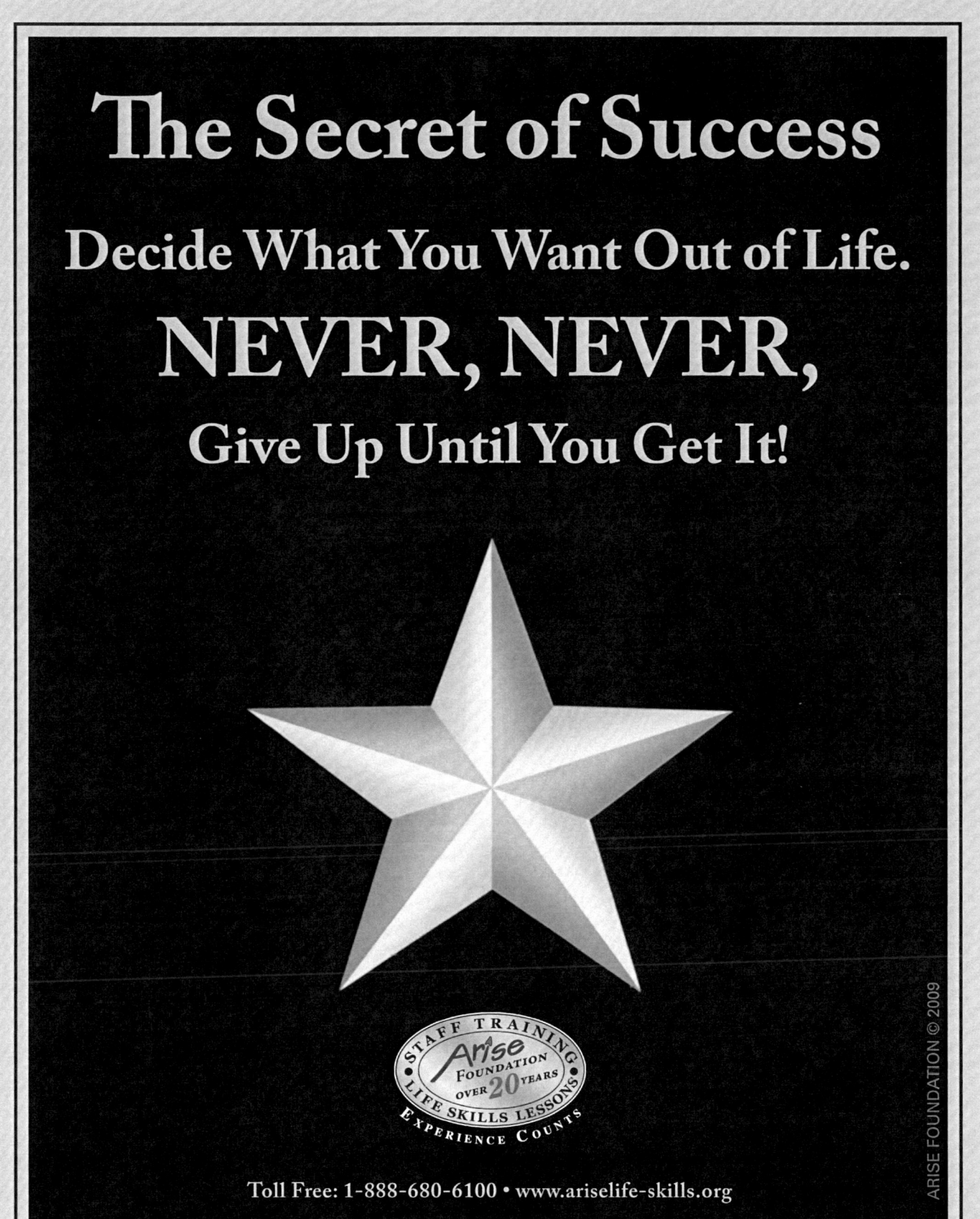

SECTION ONE
INTRODUCTION

Eating the right foods keeps you healthy. Without a nutritionally balanced diet, the body can't run properly and repair itself. America is facing an obesity epidemic. People are eating more fast food, processed food, sugar and empty calories than ever before.

What is a healthy meal? Do you need to have lots of carbohydrates or plenty of vegetables or both? Just like you need to maintain your car by changing the oil and pumping gasoline, you have to give yourself certain things to keep in good shape: vitamins, minerals, fiber, water and a variety of healthy foods are the body's fuel.

The goal for learners in this section is:

To learn about food and nutrition in order to choose a healthy diet, and avoid diseases and eating disorders.

REMEMBER TO INCLUDE THE WONDERFUL INTERACTIVE RESOURCE MATERIAL BEGINNING ON PAGE 115 AS PART OF THIS EXCITING LEARNING EXPERIENCE.

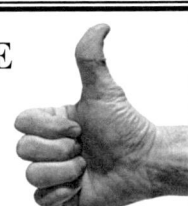

INFORM LEARNERS:
THERE WILL BE A QUIZ FOLLOWING EACH SECTION. IF THEY DON'T KNOW A WORD, ASK THEM TO REFER TO THE VOCABULARY LIST ON PAGES 98 AND 99 OF THIS MANUAL AND PAGES 67 AND 68 OF THE LEARNER'S WORKBOOK.

1 EATING WELL

A BALANCED DIET
Worksheet: *Pages 37 and 38* **Learner's Workbook:** *Pages 4 and 5*

1. Ask learners, What is a major cause of illness? Accept all responses. Do they feel better when they eat three meals a day or just once a day? What about eating fast food instead of a homemade sandwich?

2. Divide learners into groups. Each group will prepare a presentation about a balanced diet. Have them use the material on worksheet page 37 and page 4 of the Learner's Workbook. Assign each member of the group a different part. There will be three narrators, a person playing carbohydrates, someone playing protein, a person playing fats and oils, a person to play vitamins and minerals, and someone playing fiber. (The order of the presentation depends on what the group decides.) Have each group present their work.

3. On the board or a large piece of paper, write the following headings: "Carbohydrates," "Protein," "Fats and Oils," "Vitamins and Minerals," and "Fiber." Ask the learners what goes under each heading. Have them refer to the Balanced Diet worksheet.

4. Complete the Word Search on worksheet page 38 of this manual and page 5 of the Learner's Workbook and share their answers. (Answers are on page 101 of this manual.)

WHAT DO YOU KNOW? FOOD CATEGORIES; FOOD FACTS
Worksheet: *Pages 39 and 40* **Learner's Workbook:** *Pages 6 and 7*

1. Have learners complete worksheet page 39 of this manual and page 6 of the Learner's Workbook. Then, check answers with the whole group. (Answers are on page 101 of this manual.) Assure them that this is not a test, just an interesting way to give them information many people don't have. They can refer to page 37 of this manual and page 4 of the Learner's Workbook for help.

2. Give everyone a copy of page 40 of this manual and page 7 of the Learner's Workbook. Then, read each of the statements to them. Have learners respond out loud as they mark their worksheets. (Answers are on page 101 of this manual.)

3. Ask learners to share information they learned today that they didn't know.

NUTRITIONAL I.Q. QUIZ
Worksheet: *Page 41* **Learner's Workbook:** *Page 8*

Have volunteers take turns reading out loud the questions on page 41 of this manual and page 8 of the Learner's Workbook. Ask learners to write the correct answers and then discuss them as a group. (Answers are on page 102 of this manual.)

BENEFITS OF HEALTHY FOOD
Worksheet: *Page 42* **Learner's Workbook:** *Page 9*

Have learners complete page 42 of this manual and page 9 of the Learner's Workbook. Share work as a group. (Answers are on page 102 of this manual.)

WHAT'S FOR DINNER?
Worksheet: *Page 43* **Learner's Workbook:** *Page 10*

1. Discuss with learners what a healthy meal should include (fresh or frozen vegetables and fruits, dairy products [milk, yogurt, or cheese], grains [breads, pasta, or rice], and a small amount of nonfatty fish, meat, or poultry). Then, ask them to use page 43 of this manual and page 10 of the Learner's Workbook to design a nutritious dinner. They can draw a picture of it or describe it in words.

2. Have learners share their ideas for a nutritious meal.

WRAP-UP
Worksheet: *None*

Ask learners to tell you something they learned about food that they didn't know before. Write responses so that everyone can see and review them with the group.

"In health there is freedom. Health is the first of all liberties."
—Henri Frederic Amiel

2   FOOD FACTS

WATER CHECK
Worksheet: *Page 44*   **Learner's Workbook:** *Page 11*

Explain that drinking water is very important for good health. Most people don't get enough. Ask learners how much they think we should have every day. We should try to drink eight 8-oz. glasses each day to get rid of toxins and impurities from our system. Read the health benefits of drinking water on the bottom of worksheet page 44, Learner's Workbook page 11. Ask if any of the benefits surprised them. Have learners use the charts at the top of the page to keep track of how much water they drink for four days. Compare answers as a group after the exercise.

SODIUM MEANS SALT
Worksheet: *Page 45*   **Learner's Workbook:** *Page 12*

1. Have a volunteer read each statement at the top of page 45 of this manual and page 12 of the Learner's Workbook out loud to the class. Then, ask the following questions: What foods contain a lot of salt? *(chips, French fries, popcorn)* What salty foods did you eat yesterday? What disease is caused in part by eating too much salt? *(high blood pressure)*

2. On the bottom half of the page, ask them to try to match the foods with their correct sodium content. Go over the answers (found on page 102 of this manual). Did anyone guess right? Assure them that most people don't know these facts and are surprised to learn them. Ask learners, If you ate a hamburger for lunch, how much sodium can you eat for the rest of the day? *(2400mg - 875mg = 1525mg more for the day)*

TOO MUCH SUGAR
Worksheet: *Pages 46 and 47*   **Learner's Workbook:** *Pages 13 and 14*

1. Read page 46 of this manual, Learner's Workbook page 13 to the learners and explain that there are many different names for sugar. Go over the example label and point out the sugars in that food item.

2. Have the learners open to page 47 of this manual, Learner's Workbook page 14 and circle all the foods that they think have sugar *(all of them have sugar)*. Put a star next to the ones that have the most sugar *(soda, candy, ice cream, cake)*. Discuss answers as a group.

CHOICES: HEALTHY AND UNHEALTHY
Worksheet: *Page 48* **Learner's Workbook:** *Page 15*

1. Have learners open to worksheet page 48 and Learner's Workbook page 15. Ask learners what their favorite foods are. Every time they mention a "junk" food like potato chips, cookies, ice cream, cake, or soda, have them write it in the "unhealthy choice" column. When the group names healthy foods such as fruits, vegetables and grains, tell them to list these under the "healthy choice" side.

2. Write the heading "junk food" where everyone can see. Under the heading, learners will list food that is high in fat, sugar and salt *(chips, ice cream, etc.)*. Have them look at their unhealthy food choices from the activity above. Write them under the "junk food." Ask if they're eating too much junk food.

READING FOOD LABELS
Worksheet: *Pages 49 and 50* **Learner's Workbook:** *Pages 16 and 17*

1. Inform them that any food in a can, bottle, or box comes with a label that lists the food's nutrition facts. Nutrition labels let you know how the food fits into a daily diet; the amount of fat, calories, sodium, cholesterol and nutrients in that food and whether it is low-fat or fat-free. Also, tell them that ingredients are listed by weight. For instance, if the label reads "water, sugar, salt," you know that this product has more water than it does salt; in fact, water is the main ingredient.

2. Go over the food labels on page 49 of this manual and page 16 of the Learner's Workbook as a group. Ask, Which item has a lot of salt? Fat? What is each food's main ingredient? *(the first ingredient)*

3. Divide the group into pairs. Have each pair complete page 50 of this manual and page 17 of the Learner's Workbook. When they have finished, ask partners to exchange worksheets and review answers. (Answers are on page 102 of this manual.)

GROCERY RECEIPT
Worksheet: *Pages 51 and 52* **Learner's Workbook:** *Pages 18 and 19*

Have learners answer the questions on page 52 of this manual and page 19 of the Learner's Workbook, using the information on page 51 of this manual and page 18 of the Learner's Workbook. Review answers as a group when everyone has finished. (Answers are on page 102 of this manual.)

WRAP-UP
Worksheet: *None*

After learning how to be more focused on healthier food, have two volunteers act out a scene where one is ordering from a menu in a restaurant and the other person is a waiter who suggests pasta with cream sauce, fried chicken and baked fish with steamed vegetables. What should the customer order? Does the audience agree with what he picked? What would they have done differently?

3 EATING DISORDERS

EATING DISORDERS
Worksheet: *Page 53* **Learner's Workbook:** *Page 20*

Have someone read numbers 1 and 2 out loud on page 53 of this manual and page 20 of the Learner's Workbook. Then, have volunteers pick numbers 3, 4, or 5 to read and discuss each one. Ask, Does anyone know someone with these problems? Which disorder involves throwing up after eating? Which disorder involves a distorted body image and an intense fear of being fat?

DIETING QUIZ
Worksheet: *Page 54* **Learner's Workbook:** *Page 21*

Have the group take the Dieting Quiz on page 54 of this manual and page 21 of the Learner's Workbook. Then, read each question out loud and call on learners for their answers. (Answers are on page 103 of this manual.)

EATING PROBLEM
Worksheet: *Page 55* **Learner's Workbook:** *Page 22*

1. Have learners complete page 55 of this manual and page 22 of the Learner's Workbook. Explain that these questions and answers can serve as a guide to let us know if someone has problems with eating.

2. Ask how many answered "yes" to three or more questions. Then, ask them to write down on a piece of paper what they think their problem with eating is. If you answered yes to many of the questions, speak to a trusted adult for help. Read the statistics below to learners.

- An estimated 1 in 100 American women binges and purges to lose weight.
- 15 percent of young women have significantly disordered eating attitudes and behavior.
- An estimated 1 in 3 of all dieters develop compulsive dieting attitudes and behaviors.
- Of these, one quarter will develop full or partial eating disorders.
- Each day Americans spend an average of $109 million on dieting and diet related products.
  (source: http://www.annecollins.com)

WHAT I THINK OF MY BODY
Worksheet: *Page 56* **Learner's Workbook:** *Page 23*

1. Ask learners what they would change about their bodies if they could. Would they get a nose job? Lose weight? Explain that most people are never happy with the way they look; not even the most beautiful movie stars feel they are perfect. This type of thinking is one cause of eating disorders.

2. Have them complete page 56 of this manual and page 23 of the Learner's Workbook.

DANGER SIGNS
Worksheet: *Page 57* **Learner's Workbook:** *Page 24*

Ask, What are the signs of eating disorders? *(weight loss, complaining about weight, constant trips to the bathroom after meals, never eating in front of anyone)* Write responses where everyone can see, then distribute page 57 of this manual and page 24 of the Learner's Workbook for them to complete. (Answers are on page 103 of this manual.)

ATTITUDE CHANGES
Worksheet: *Page 58* **Learner's Workbook:** *Page 25*

1. Have a volunteer read page 58 of this manual and page 25 of the Learner's Workbook out loud. Ask learners what they think of these statements. Discuss their opinions as a group.

2. Divide the group into pairs. Then, encourage them to write down ways that they could change attitudes that contribute to eating disorders. Have partners read their ideas out loud to the rest of the group. Answers may include *concentrating on people's good qualities, not how much they weigh; realizing that advertising is only about selling products and making people spend more; knowing that people in magazines and movies don't look perfect all the time, and it is unrealistic to try to look like them.*

WRAP-UP
Worksheet: *None*

Ask them if they can take charge of their bodies now with the information they have learned. How do they plan to do this?

COMPLETE THE REVIEW ACTIVITY.
THEN IT'S QUIZ TIME! THE SECTION ONE QUIZ IS ON PAGE 107.
THE ANSWERS ARE ON PAGE 114.

REVIEW ACTIVITY: FACT OR FICTION?

Ask learners the following questions out loud.

1. A hot dog has 875 grams of sodium. (Fact)

2. Sodium is used to preserve food. (Fact)

3. Food companies do not list sodium on the food label. (Fiction)

4. Foods ending in "-ose" contain sugar. (Fact)

5. Sugar is a major source of calories, but not vitamins or minerals. (Fact)

6. Eating sweets makes you hungry. (Fact)

7. People with anorexia have a realistic body image. (Fiction)

8. A compulsive eater eats all the time. (Fact)

9. A 12-ounce bottle of soda has six teaspoons of sugar. (Fiction—it has 10 teaspoons)

10. Foods high in fat can make you gain weight and lead to serious illnesses. (Fact)

SECTION TWO
INTRODUCTION

MyPlace outlines what and how much we should eat to stay healthy. By studying it, we can see the proteins, carbohydrates, fiber, minerals, fats, and vitamins that we need every day. Eating a balanced diet is important for good health. MyPlace is a handy guide to help you make good food choices each day. Use it to help plan meals.

By using MyPlace and eating fresh fruit, vegetables, lean meats, low-fat milk products and whole grains, you will look and feel great.

The goal for learners in this section is:

To be able to select healthy foods in order to become a fit, healthy and attractive human being.

REMEMBER TO INCLUDE THE WONDERFUL INTERACTIVE RESOURCE MATERIAL BEGINNING ON PAGE 115 AS PART OF THIS EXCITING LEARNING EXPERIENCE.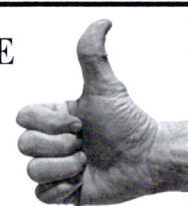

INFORM LEARNERS:
THERE WILL BE A QUIZ FOLLOWING EACH SECTION.
IF THEY DON'T KNOW A WORD, ASK THEM TO REFER TO THE VOCABULARY LIST ON PAGES 98 AND 99 OF THIS MANUAL AND PAGES 67 AND 68 OF THE LEARNER'S WORKBOOK.

1   MYPLACE

UNDERSTANDING MYPLACE; THE RIGHT CHOICES

Worksheet: *Pages 59 and 60*   **Learner's Workbook:** *Pages 26 and 27*

1. Have learners open to worksheet pages 59 and 60 and Learner's Workbook pages 26 and 27, Understanding MyPlace. Ask learners to look at the information on worksheet page 60 and Learner's Workbook page 26. Call on volunteers to read the two pages out loud. Ask, How many ounces of grains should you eat each day? *(6)* From what group should you eat the least? *(fats/oils)* How many cups of fruits and vegetables combined should you eat in a day? *(4.5 cups)* Should you eat foods from all the different fruit groups? *(yes)* Have learners tell you some food choices for a healthy breakfast, lunch and dinner. Ask them if they think they are eating healthy foods every day.

2. Have learners look back at the grocery receipt on worksheet page 51, Learner's Workbook page 18. Using what they know about healthy food choices, have them circle the items that are good choices. Why did they pick those items? Which items on the list are unhealthy choices? Why?

A RACE AGAINST TIME

Worksheet: *Page 61*   **Learner's Workbook:** *Page 28*

1. Open to page 61 of this manual and page 28 of the Learner's Workbook. In small groups, learners will think of a healthy food beginning with each letter of the alphabet. Provide some examples, such as apples for A, broccoli for B. Learners can get creative with X and Z, such as "x-tra lean meats." At the end of five minutes, everyone must stop writing.

2. Review answers together. Each correct one receives a point. The person with the most points wins.

THE BLANK MYPLATE

Worksheet: *Page 62*   **Learner's Workbook:** *Page 29*

Have them complete the blank pyramid on page 62 of this manual and page 29 of the Learner's Workbook. They may use the information on worksheet pages 59 and 60, Learner's Workbook pages 26 and 27 and draw or write the names of the foods. Encourage creativity. When everyone has finished, display their work for the group.

PLANNING MEALS

Worksheet: *Page 63*   **Learner's Workbook:** *Page 30*

1. Divide learners into small groups. Have each plan two menus on page 63 of this manual and page 30 of the Learner's Workbook—one with smart meal choices, such as cereal and skim milk for breakfast, and the other with less healthy ones, such as sausage and donuts.

2. Ask them to share their papers with everyone. Which of these will keep them alive and healthy for a long time?

3. Instruct learners to design a menu for one meal that includes at least one serving of food from each food group. The menus must include a main dish and at least one side dish and a beverage.

MAKING CHANGES

Worksheet: *Page 64*   **Learner's Workbook:** *Page 31*

1. Encourage everyone to discuss what they eat every day. Have learners look at MyPlace to see if they're following a healthy diet or if they need to make changes. Are they having cake for breakfast and doughnuts with a soda for lunch? Is this a good idea? Why or why not?

2. Direct all to complete page 64 of this manual and page 31 of the Learner's Workbook. Ask them if they think they could live with some healthy changes. Why? Why not?

FAVORITE FOODS

Worksheet: *Page 65*   **Learner's Workbook:** *Page 32*

1. Instruct learners to turn to worksheet page 65, Learner's Workbook page 32. Ask them to list their favorite foods in each category. Is there one missing? *(fats, sweets)*

2. Tell everyone to brainstorm substitutes for foods like ice cream and burgers. Answers may include *low-fat frozen yogurt, fruit, and grilled chicken.*

WRAP-UP

Worksheet: *None*

Have each person draw a cartoon—for young kids—of a vegetable with a face and clothes. They should give their character a name and write a message about eating healthy. Share their artwork as a group.

2 NUTRIENTS I

TYPES OF NUTRIENTS
Worksheet: *Page 66*   **Learner's Workbook:** *Page 33*

1. Explain that there are more than 50 nutrients, which are divided into several groups: macronutrients like proteins, carbohydrates, and fats; micronutrients like vitamins and minerals; water and fiber. List these on the board or a large piece of paper. Our bodies need these in order to have energy to get up in the morning, stay healthy and live a long life.

2. Give each person a copy of page 66 of this manual and page 33 of the Learner's Workbook, explaining that the answers can be found in the word bank at the bottom of the page. Then, go through each item with them, calling on volunteers for the answers. (Answers are on page 103 of this manual.)

SEARCH FOR PROTEIN
Worksheet: *Page 67*   **Learner's Workbook:** *Page 34*

1. Inform learners that proteins are foods that help us grow and heal our bodies. They include beef, pork, chicken, turkey, fish, eggs, and beans. Other products, such as grains, nuts and vegetables, also contain some protein.

2. Ask the group to circle the protein-rich foods on page 67 of this manual and page 34 of the Learner's Workbook. (Answers are on page 103 of this manual.)

CHEER FOR PROTEIN
Worksheet: *Page 68*   **Learner's Workbook:** *Page 35*

Have volunteers jump read page 68 of this manual or page 35 of the Learner's Workbook. (Jump reading begins by having one learner read until the end of a sentence or idea. Another learner jumps in and continues to read until the end of another sentence or thought. This continues until all the information has been read.) Discuss the importance of proteins and foods that contain them. Have learners write a short summary of the types of proteins people need to eat to maintain their health.

ALL ABOUT CARBOHYDRATES
Worksheet: *Page 69*   **Learner's Workbook:** *Page 36*

1. Tell the group they will be learning about carbohydrates next. Explain that they provide energy for our bodies, but if we have too many, they will be converted and stored as fat. (All carbohydrates turn into sugar in the body.)

2. Using page 69 of this manual or page 36 of the Learner's Workbook, have different volunteers read the information in each shape out loud. Go over any questions they may have.

CARBO FUEL; THUMBS UP/THUMBS DOWN
Worksheet: *Pages 70 and 71*   **Learner's Workbook:** *Pages 37 and 38*

1. Inform learners that there are complex carbohydrates (made up of two or more simple sugars linked together and found in grains, fruits, legumes [peas and beans] and other vegetables) and simple carbohydrates (sometimes called simple sugars, including fructose [fruit sugar], sucrose [table sugar], and lactose [milk sugar], as well as several other sugars). Read the items on the worksheet page 70, Learner's Workbook page 37 out loud and direct learners to put a circle around complex carbohydrates and an X on the simple carbohydrates. (Answers are on page 104 of this manual.) Explain to learners that it is healthier to eat more complex carbohydrates than simple ones.

2. Have everyone complete page 71 of this manual or page 38 of the Learner's Workbook. Then have each read their entries out loud to the group. *(Thumbs down may include sugary cereals, donuts, cookies, and cake.)*

ALL ABOUT FIBER
Worksheet: *Page 72*   **Learner's Workbook:** *Page 39*

1. Tell learners that there are two types of fiber. One is "soluble" *(sol-yoo-bul)*. It helps reduce cholesterol and is found in oats and beans. The other is "unsoluble" and is found in fruit, wheat, whole grains, and popcorn. List the following two facts where everyone can see: (1) Fiber is not digested, but helps move food through the body. (2) In order to stay healthy, we must eat 20 to 30 grams of it a day.

2. Make sure everyone has a copy of page 72 of this manual and page 39 of the Learner's Workbook and instruct them to complete it.

WRAP-UP
Worksheet: *None*

Ask a volunteer to pretend he is teaching a nutrition lesson to second graders. What would he say about carbohydrates, sugar and fiber?

Nutrients II

Vitamin Web

Worksheet: *Page 73* **Learner's Workbook:** *Page 40*

1. Ask learners if they know how to get their needed vitamins. Do you get them from drinking water or soda? How about eating French fries? Accept all responses. Tell them that the best way is by eating healthy food. "Lycopene" *(lie-ko-peen)*, for example, which is found in tomatoes, helps the body fight certain cancers. If you eat a healthy, balanced diet, you don't need to buy vitamin pills.

2. Complete page 73 of this manual or page 40 of the Learner's Workbook as a group, writing answers where everyone can see. Have learners copy them onto their worksheets. Use the answer sheet to help when they don't know the answers. (Answers are on page 104 of this manual.)

3. Test their understanding of the information. Ask, What does Vitamin C do? How about Vitamin D?

Vitamins and Minerals in Your Diet

Worksheet: *Pages 74 and 75* **Learner's Workbook:** *Pages 41 and 42*

1. Encourage learners to discuss what they know about the importance of vitamins in a healthy diet.

2. Have a volunteer read page 74 of this manual and page 41 of the Learner's Workbook. Ask the group to fill out the worksheet, using the information they read.

3. Have learners turn to worksheet page 75, Learner's Workbook page 42. Ask them to get into pairs to read and discuss the worksheet.

4. Ask learners the following questions:
   a. What mineral builds strong bones and teeth? (calcium)
   b. What mineral is found in red meat and chicken? (iron)
   c. What mineral builds healthy blood? (iron)
   d. What mineral is found in beans? (iron)
   e. What mineral is found in cheese? (calcium)
   f. What mineral protects the heart by smoothing artery walls? (calcium)

RESTAURANT MENUS AND MINERALS
Worksheet: *Page 76* **Learner's Workbook:** *Page 43*

1. Explain that calcium and iron are minerals (natural substances) needed for healthy bones and teeth, and to give us energy. Have learners use page 76 of this manual and page 43 of the Learner's Workbook to choose foods that contain iron and calcium *(all the foods listed are high in calcium or iron)*.

2. Choose several volunteers to role-play being on a dinner date and ordering foods from menu 1 or 2.

FACTS ABOUT FAT
Worksheet: *Page 77* **Learner's Workbook:** *Page 44*

Ask learners to read the paragraph on page 77 of this manual and page 44 of the Learner's Workbook and then answer the true or false questions at the bottom. Once everyone has finished, review their work. (Answers are on page 104 of this manual.)

FAT MAKES FAT COMIC STRIP
Worksheet: *Page 78* **Learner's Workbook:** *Page 45*

1. Explain that when eating foods high in fat, we transfer *animal fat* into our own bodies. Too much saturated fat (animal fat), or cholesterol, clogs up our arteries, which can lead to heart problems. It's important to read food labels and avoid fatty foods. (For example, *many processed foods like bologna, hot dogs, and sausage are often high in fat*.)

2. Have learners read the top of worksheet page 78, Learner's Workbook page 45.

3. Then have learners create a comic strip showing someone eating low-fat foods on the bottom of page 78 of this manual and page 45 of the Learner's Workbook. Display their artwork for all to see.

WRAP-UP
Worksheet: *None*

Ask them to tell you what they will order next time they go out to eat. Is it really healthy and full of vitamins and minerals or not? Discuss their opinions about this topic.

COMPLETE THE REVIEW ACTIVITY.
THEN, IT'S QUIZ TIME! THE SECTION TWO QUIZ IS ON PAGE 108
AND THE ANSWERS ARE ON PAGE 114.

REVIEW ACTIVITY

Tell learners that they are now going to complete the crossword puzzle below based on the nutrition lessons they learned in section two.

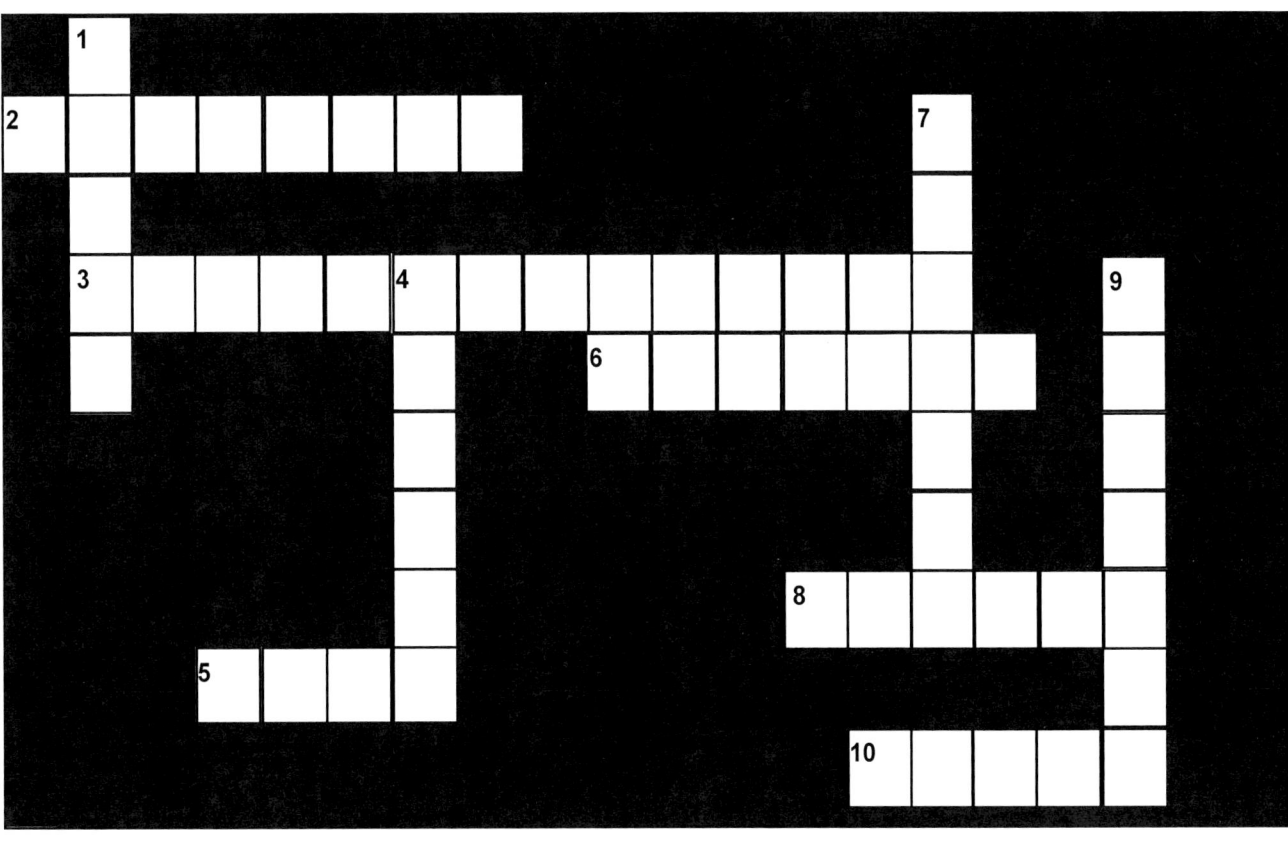

ACROSS

2. _____ help you stay healthy. Some examples are A, E, C and D.

3. If you are constantly worried about getting fat, you might have an _____.

5. _____ and oils make you overweight and can give you heart problems.

6. Iron is a _____.

8. _____ is another word for salt.

10. Calcium helps you build strong teeth and _____.

DOWN

1. ____ helps you digest food.

4. Whole ____ are better for you. Some examples are whole wheat, brown rice and oats.

7. The Food _____ gives you an idea of what sorts of foods you should eat each day.

9. Beans and peas are also called _____.

ARISE Basic Health 101: Nutrition and Exercise, Instructor's Manual, Page 25

SECTION THREE
INTRODUCTION

Not all of us realize that there is more than one type of fitness. It's possible for someone to be in good shape physically, but still need to work on flexibility and strength. Even the most muscular, fit person may be completely inflexible.

Because cardiovascular (heart) fitness is different from health-related and sports fitness, there are several forms of exercise we need to learn. It's interesting to know that each one brings with it different benefits.

REMEMBER TO INCLUDE THE WONDERFUL INTERACTIVE RESOURCE MATERIAL BEGINNING ON PAGE 115 AS PART OF THIS EXCITING LEARNING EXPERIENCE.

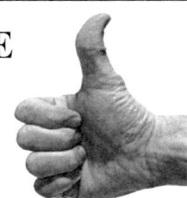

The goal for learners in this section is:

To understand how important exercise is in our daily lives and how it helps us live longer and healthier.

INFORM LEARNERS:
IF THEY DON'T KNOW A WORD, ASK THEM TO REFER TO THE VOCABULARY LIST ON PAGES 98 AND 99 OF THIS MANUAL AND PAGES 67 AND 68 OF THE LEARNER'S WORKBOOK.

1 BEING PHYSICALLY FIT

DEFINING PHYSICAL FITNESS; MY OWN PHYSICAL FITNESS
Worksheet: *Pages 79 and 80*   **Learner's Workbook:** *Pages 46 and 47*

1. Ask learners what physical fitness means to them. Allow the group to respond. Have a volunteer read the definition on page 79 of this manual and page 46 of the Learner's Workbook. Then, ask if they know what the terms "health-related" and "sports-related" fitness mean. Then, read the definitions on the worksheet.

2. On page 80 of this manual and page 47 of the Learner's Workbook, direct everyone to write about their favorite physical activities and how often they do them. Answers may include *weightlifting, playing basketball, running, and cycling.* Share their answers as a group.

COMPONENTS OF PHYSICAL FITNESS
Worksheet: *Page 81*   **Learner's Workbook:** *Page 48*

1. Inform learners that people exercise to be healthy or to perform well at a sport. Have learners turn to worksheet page 81 and Learner's Workbook page 48. Encourage everyone to indicate which points are the most important to health and sports-related fitness. If they feel that an item doesn't matter to either one, tell them to mark it with a zero. (All are related to sports and health.)

2. After everyone has finished, review worksheets as a group.

OPINION ACTIVITY
Worksheet: *None*

1. Ask, What will you do to improve your fitness levels? Do you plan to start exercising more? Eating healthier food? What changes will you make in your life? Discuss their opinions and thoughts.

2. Encourage learners to consider this: If you could switch bodies with any famous athlete or celebrity, who would you be? Why did you choose that person?

3. Have each person give a two-minute presentation on his favorite sport and the importance of doing physical activity.

CARDIOVASCULAR FITNESS—IN YOUR OWN WORDS

Worksheet: *Page 82* **Learner's Workbook:** *Page 49*

Ask for six volunteers to each read one sentence out loud from worksheet page 82 or page 49 of the Learner's Workbook. After each one reads his sentence, have him call on one of the other learners to repeat, in his own words, what it means. Do this with all.

DESIGN AN EXERCISE ROUTINE

Worksheet: *Page 83* **Learner's Workbook:** *Page 50*

1. Have everyone brainstorm why being fit helps them feel better. Answers may include *more energy, better flexibility, and less fat.*

2. Instruct each person to pretend they are the coach of a sports team about to play in a championship game. On worksheet page 83 and page 50 of the Learner's Workbook, encourage them to design an exercise routine for a week. Share answers as a group.

WRAP-UP

Worksheet: *None*

Discuss what new information they learned about physical fitness in this section that they didn't know before. What did they find most interesting? Share their opinions and thoughts.

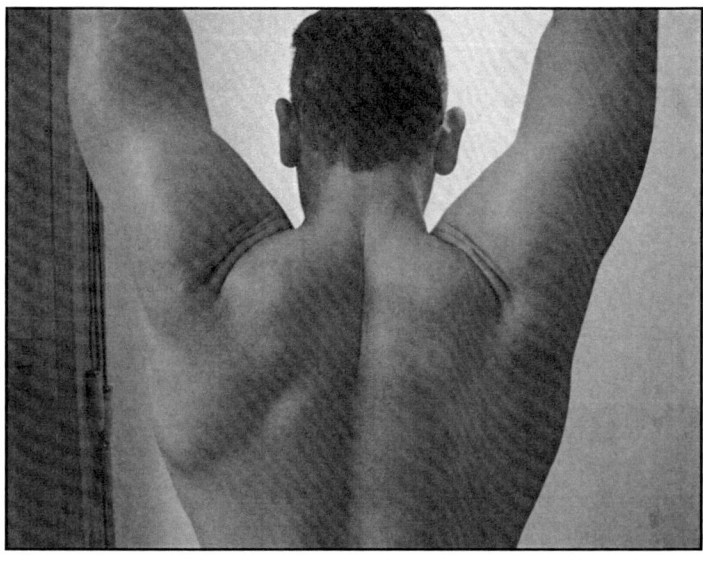

DISCUSS THE FOLLOWING AS A GROUP:

Did you know that there are 639 muscles in the body, each with its own name?

—*The Big Book of Tell Me Why*

2   EXERCISE

FACTS AND BENEFITS: TRUE OR FALSE QUIZ
Worksheet: *Page 84*   **Learner's Workbook:** *Page 51*

1. Explain that although most people are familiar with the benefits of exercise, they also have a good deal of wrong information.

2. Ask each person to state why they think jogging or playing sports is good for them. Write their comments where everyone can see. *(Exercise helps us maintain our ideal weight; it keeps the heart healthy and pumped full of oxygenated blood; it strengthens the lungs and muscles.)*

3. Have everyone test his knowledge by completing page 84 of this manual and page 51 of the Learner's Workbook. Then ask if group members can think of anything else to add. (Answers are on page 104 of this manual.)

EXERCISE IS GOOD FOR EVERYTHING
Worksheet: *Page 85*   **Learner's Workbook:** *Page 52*

1. Ask if learners know anyone who is overweight and doesn't exercise. What would you tell them about the benefits of exercising?

2. Direct a volunteer to read page 85 of this manual and page 52 of the Learner's Workbook. Then, have them use the space provided on the worksheet to write a letter to someone they know asking him to exercise and explaining why it is so important.

WAYS TO EXERCISE
Worksheet: *Page 86*   **Learner's Workbook:** *Page 53*

Divide learners into small groups. Encourage them to brainstorm their favorite types of exercise, and list these on page 86 of this manual and page 53 of the Learner's Workbook. Go around the room and have everyone share what they wrote and why. Make sure they talk about the type of equipment they need for each exercise and any rules they need to follow.

WALKING MAP
Worksheet: *Page 87* **Learner's Workbook:** *Page 54*

1. Ask for a volunteer to read the tips on page 87 of this manual and page 54 of the Learner's Workbook. After each statement, discuss it with the group. Do learners think these suggestions are good? Would they rather go to the gym or work out at home? Why or why not?

2. Have everyone make a map of his own neighborhood. Are there places they can walk to? How about to the grocery store or a friend's house?

EXCUSES
Worksheet: *None*

1. Ask, Does everyone here exercise every day? Why? Why not? They may have many reasons why they don't. List these where everyone can see. Answers may include *I get home too late; I don't have time; I'm always too tired; I don't have money for a gym membership or exercise equipment.*

2. Challenge the group to brainstorm practical solutions for these and any other problems mentioned by everyone: *Do sit-ups in the morning before leaving; Work out for just 10 minutes; If you jog, you will have more energy and not feel so tired; Walking is free.*

THE PLEDGE TO EXERCISE
Worksheet: *Page 88* **Learner's Workbook:** *Page 55*

1. Tell learners that we must all plan for exercise or we won't do it. It's hard to get up an hour earlier three times a week, but it will pay off.

2. Have volunteers take turns reading the Pledge to Exercise on page 88 of this manual and page 55 of the Learner's Workbook. Have them sign their names.

WRAP-UP
Worksheet: *None*

What are some of the benefits of exercise? Write answers where everyone can see. Then, ask what type of exercise most appeals to each of them and why. Does everyone agree on the benefits? Why? Why not?

3 FLEXIBILITY AND STRENGTH

DEFINING FLEXIBILITY

Worksheet: *Page 89*   **Learner's Workbook:** *Page 56*

1. Ask learners to define "flexibility." Accept all answers. *(ability to move the body through a full range of motion.)*

2. Instruct them to refer to page 89 of this manual and page 56 of the Learner's Workbook. Call on a volunteer to read out loud. Do they think running or rollerskating might help? Why or why not? Ask for a demonstration.

WORKING AT FLEXIBILITY

Worksheet: *Pages 90-93*   **Learner's Workbook:** *Pages 57-60*

1. Give each person copies of pages 90-93 of this manual or pages 57-60 of the Learner's Workbook. Ask the learners to study the exercises for a few minutes.

2. Have six volunteers try each of the exercises on the worksheet page 90, Learner's Workbook page 57. When finished, ask them how they felt doing these. Also encourage others to ask questions.

3. Ask the learners to take home the worksheets and try all the exercises, including the yoga poses. When they return, ask them what they thought of the exercises. How did they feel afterwards? If there is time, do all of the exercises during the group session.

FLEXIBILITY TRAINING PRINCIPLES

Worksheet: *Page 94*   **Learner's Workbook:** *Page 61*

1. Have four volunteers each read one of the sections on page 94 of this manual and page 61 of the Learner's Workbook. Then, ask the group if they are willing to do the flexibility exercises three times a week for at least four weeks.

2. Ask learners how they will plan a workout time and place. Help them write a schedule. Answers may include *in your living room at 6 a.m.; in your bedroom when you get home from work or school.*

DEFINING MUSCULAR STRENGTH

Worksheet: *Page 95* **Learner's Workbook:** *Page 62*

1. Have learners brainstorm ideas about what "muscular strength" means to them. Allow for answers. Then, explain that it increases our ability to perform physical activity, reduces the chances of injury, and helps the quality of personal performance.

2. Ask for a volunteer to read page 95 of this manual and page 62 of the Learner's Workbook. Did they all understand the information? Review if necessary.

MUSCULAR STRENGTH WORD FIND

Worksheet: *Page 96* **Learner's Workbook:** *Page 63*

1. Have them complete page 96 of this manual and page 63 of the Learner's Workbook.

2. If anyone had problems finding a word, call on members of the group to share their answers. (Answers are on page 105 of this manual.)

ACTIVITY LOG

Worksheet: *Page 97* **Learner's Workbook:** *Page 64*

Direct each person to complete page 97 of this manual and page 64 of the Learner's Workbook. When everyone has finished, review them as a group. Ask, Do most of you get at least an hour of exercise a day? Are you more likely to do so in the morning, afternoon or evening? How do you think you can do more physical activity?

WRAP-UP

Worksheet: *None*

Ask, What is the difference between being flexible and being strong? Then, ask for a brief demonstration of some of the stretching exercises they learned in this section.

COMPLETE THE REVIEW ACTIVITY.
THEN IT'S QUIZ TIME! THE SECTION THREE QUIZ IS ON PAGE 109. ANSWERS ARE ON PAGE 114.

REVIEW ACTIVITY

1. Play "Review Bingo." On blank pieces of paper, have learners draw four lines separating the page into nine boxes.

2. Have learners write the following words and phrases on the board, then copy them into any box they like: exercise, physical fitness, cardiovascular fitness, walking, flexibility, muscular strength, aerobic exercise, skateboarding, stretching.

3. Ask learners to tear another piece of paper into nine small markers to be placed on a box when the word in that box is called.

4. Call out the words and phrases listed on the board. Have players tell you what they mean as they put their markers in the boxes. The first player to fill three boxes in a row—horizontally, vertically, or diagonally—wins.

Here are some possible answers for what each phrase means (excluding walking and skateboarding):

<u>Exercise</u>: moving the body to increase heart rate, build strength and increase flexibility.
<u>Physical fitness</u>: the overall condition of a person's body
<u>Cardiovascular Fitness</u>: the ability of the heart, lungs and circulatory system to provide muscles with oxygen.
<u>Flexibility</u>: ability to move joints through a full range of motion.
<u>Muscular Strength</u>: how much force your muscles can take.
<u>Aerobic Exercise</u>: exercise that increases the heart rate, such as walking, jogging, cycling, swimming, dancing, etc.
<u>Stretching</u>: moving the joints and muscles to their maximum range.

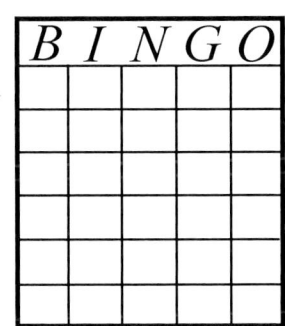

**CONGRATULATIONS! YOU HAVE FINISHED THIS BOOK.
TO MAKE SURE LEARNERS UNDERSTOOD THE MATERIAL, YOU MAY GIVE THEM THE ASSESSMENT ON PAGES 110 AND 111 OF THIS MANUAL.**

WORTH REMEMBERING

Have three volunteers read these quotes out loud and ask learners what they think each one means. This page is also located on page 65 of the Learner's Workbook.

"More die in the United States from too much food than from too little."
—*John Kenneth Galbraith, American economist*

"We are digging our graves with our teeth."
—*Thomas Moffett, American physician*

Did you know that 60 percent of the human body is water? If you could squeeze out a human being like a lemon, you would get about 11 gallons of water.

WORTH REMEMBERING (CONT.)

Have three volunteers read these quotes out loud and ask learners what they think each one means.

> **Lycopene (lie-ko-pen), which is found in tomatoes, helps the body fight certain cancers. If you eat a healthy, balanced diet, you don't need to buy vitamin pills.**

> **"Nothing lifts me out of a bad mood better than a hard workout on my treadmill. It never fails. To us, exercise is nothing short of a miracle."**
> —Cher, American actress, director, singer

> **"Exercise: you don't have time not to."**
> —Source unknown

ARISE Basic Health 101: Nutrition and Exercise

Learner's Worksheets

"He who enjoys good health is rich, though he knows it not."
— *Italian Proverb*

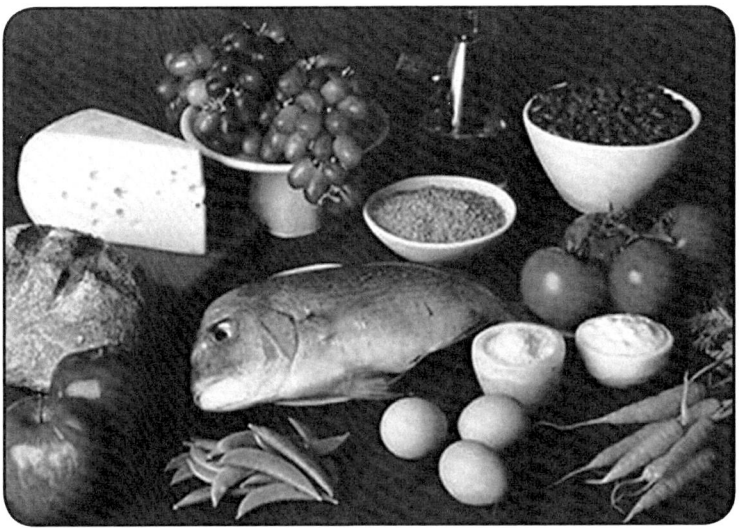

www.ariselife-skills.org

A Balanced Diet

Narrator 1: When you eat healthy foods, you have more energy and fun. You may also have more money because fresh foods generally cost less than packaged ones, and you'll save on doctor bills.

Narrator 2: Your body converts food into energy just as an automobile engine converts gasoline into energy. Use only "clean-burning" fuels, such as fresh fruits, fresh or frozen vegetables, whole grains, low-fat dairy products, low-fat meats, and small amounts of fats and oils.

Narrator 3: Whole grains include natural brown rice and whole-wheat bread; vitamins are found in citrus fruits (vitamin C), spinach (vitamin A), black beans (vitamin B1), milk (vitamin D), and almonds (vitamin E). These foods give you nutrients needed for good health because they are rich in the following:

Group 1: **Carbohydrates:** These have been the basis of nutrition throughout history. The primary sources are wheat, rice, corn, beans, potatoes, fruits, vegetables, and grains.

Group 2: **Protein:** Protein provides important materials to build and maintain muscles and other body tissues. Although many foods include this, foods that provide the most protein are meat, poultry, fish, and some dairy products.

Group 3: **Fats and Oils:** Meat, cooking and salad oils, butter, mayonnaise, whole milk, and cream are all sources of fat. A certain amount in our diet is necessary, but too much fat can be harmful. Animal fat is high in cholesterol and saturated fats, which increase the risk of heart disease. Palm oil is high in saturated fat and can clog arteries. Eating green vegetables may help keep arteries from becoming clogged with fat.

Group 4: **Vitamins and Minerals:** Minerals help build your body's systems and keep them going; vitamins help change the food you eat into energy. You receive plenty of these if you eat a well-balanced diet of natural foods. Minerals in foods include calcium (in milk and cheese) and iron (in lean red meat, some breakfast cereals, raisins, dried peaches, and some fish and poultry).

Group 5: **Fiber:** Dietary fiber is necessary to keep your digestion running smoothly. Whole grains, green vegetables, and fruits are excellent sources.

A Balanced Diet (cont.)

Find the words in the word bank. Answers can be vertical, horizontal, or diagonal.

```
D X J U E E I N I S T I U R F
F L X V V B Q C H Q C N O P S
G C Y G V V S O H E A L T H Y
P Z H Z N Y N Y A D R E R U S
S K K S O F I H U I W N C Y N
N N M Y I S E L B A T E G E V
R F I B T F T D H S E R F V H
I O E A I E O L E Y N G U E F
O R D E R R L K Y M Y H M B
T F N A T G P I L T Z M Z D V
Y R T V U L R V K F Y C F T X
I E O E N G W R C J D D Q J H
D A P X Z M F L D U Z W E M Q
```

WORD BANK

Energy   Healthy
Fiber   Nutrition
Fresh   Proteins
Fruits   Vegetables
Grains

What Do You Know? Food Categories

Match the food in the left column with its label on the right. (Most have more than one.)

Carbohydrate   Calcium
Protein   Iron
Fats/Oils   Vitamin C
Vitamin E   Vitamin A
Fiber   Vitamin D

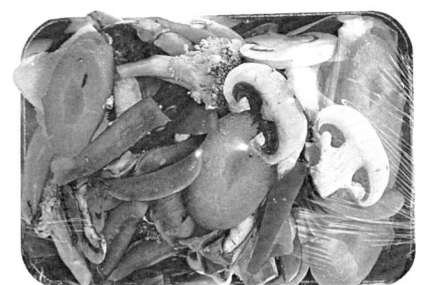

1. Brown Rice _____
2. Raisins _____
3. Spinach _____
4. Cheese _____
5. Milk _____
6. Almonds _____
7. Corn _____
8. Chicken _____
9. Beans _____
10. Oranges _____
11. Beef _____
12. Apple _____

WHAT DO YOU KNOW? FOOD FACTS

Write "T" for true or "F" for false on the line before each statement.

_____ 1. Too much salt in your diet can lead to high blood pressure.

_____ 2. Refined sugars (found in such foods as soft drinks and candy) contain no vitamins, minerals or protein.

_____ 3. Foods high in fat can make you gain too much weight and can lead to serious illnesses.

_____ 4. Carbohydrates are found in foods like rice, corn, beans, potatoes, and pasta.

_____ 5. The body needs protein as well as fat to function properly.

_____ 6. Protein is needed to build muscles. Muscles burn fat. (Exercise builds muscles.)

_____ 7. The best diet is one that has no fat, sugar, or salt in it.

_____ 8. A diet low in fat and cholesterol helps keep the arteries (the tubes your heart pumps blood through) in your heart from becoming clogged with fat.

_____ 9. The only good way to get vitamins is to take vitamin pills.

_____ 10. Whole grains are a good source of fiber.

Nutritional I.Q. Quiz

Choose the correct answer.

1. How many teaspoons of sugar are there in a 12-ounce bottle of soda?

    a. 2 teaspoons   c. 6 teaspoons
    b. 4 teaspoons   d. 10 teaspoons

2. Which of these typical fast-food items has the most sodium?

    a. Cheeseburger   c. Milkshake
    b. Apple pie   d. French fries

3. Which one has more fat and calories?

    a. Slice of cheesecake   b. Triple cheeseburger

4. An apple is a good source of fiber.

    a. True   b. False

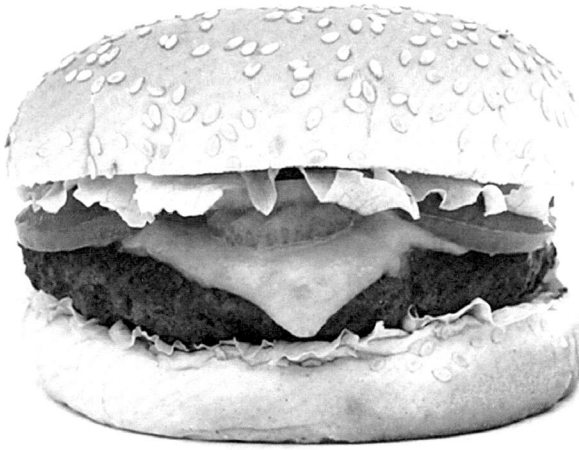

BENEFITS OF HEALTHY FOOD

Fill in the blanks with the missing vowels. Cross off the letter from the bank once you have used it.

1. Healthy foods, such as whole grains, b_ _ns, fresh fruits, and vegetables can protect you from cancer, heart disease, high blood pressure, diabetes, and many other diseases. Friendly foods are low in fat, salt, and s_g_r. They are high in fiber.

2. These foods are as good for your mind and _m_t_ _ns as they are for your body. They help you focus your m_nt_l attention and avoid fatigue. They can even help free you from the frustrated feelings that can lead to _v_r_ _t_ng.

3. A diet of friendly foods costs about a third less than the typical _m_r_c_n diet. When you eat n_t_r_l foods, you also save money because you experience fewer sick days and don't spend as much on doctors and prescriptions.

4. Learning, m_m_r_, and intelligence are all controlled by chemicals that carry messages in the brain.

5. They influence your I.Q., wake you up, put you to sleep, make you happy, sad, or calm, control your _pp_t_t_, dreams, coordination, and sex drive. The level of chemicals in your br_ _n is controlled by the foods you eat.

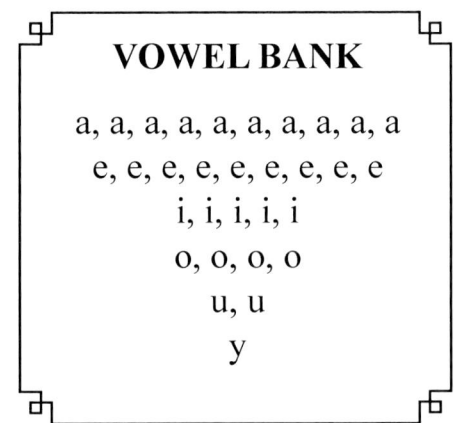

VOWEL BANK

a, a, a, a, a, a, a, a, a, a
e, e, e, e, e, e, e, e, e
i, i, i, i, i
o, o, o, o
u, u
y

WHAT'S FOR DINNER?

Draw a healthy meal. Not all of us are born artists. Do the best you can to satisfy yourself.

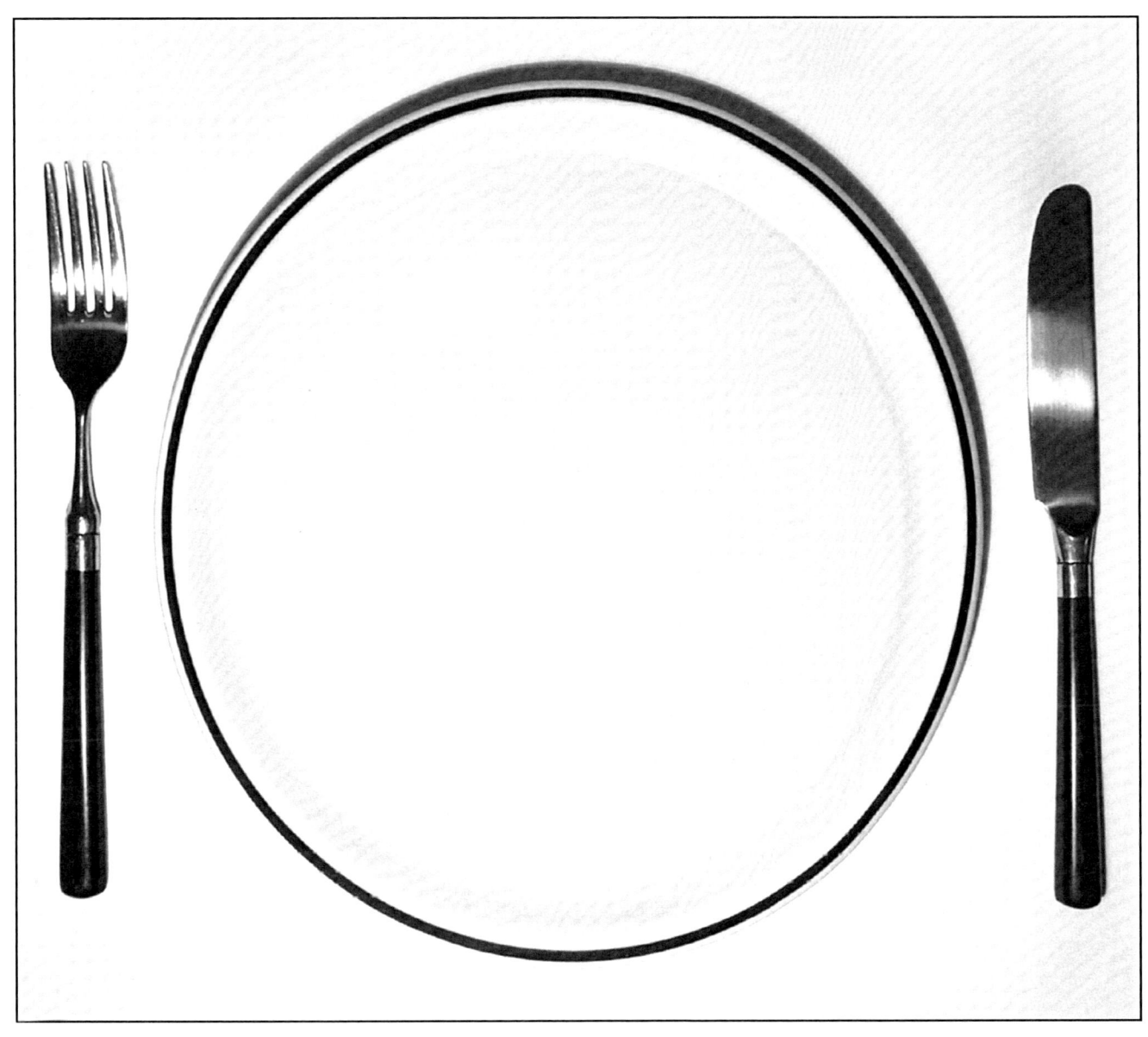

WATER CHECK

For the next few days, keep track of how much water you drink. Every time you have an eight-ounce glass of water, cross out one of the pictures below.

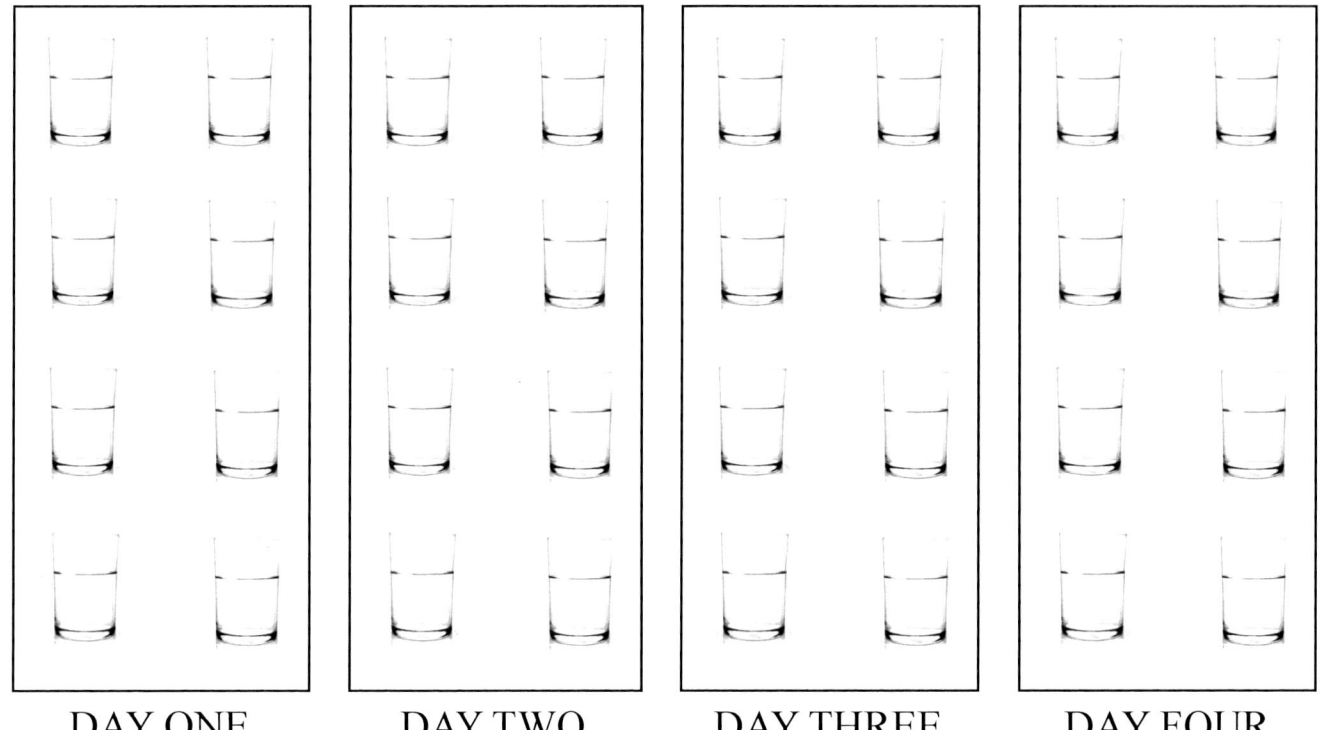

DAY ONE   DAY TWO   DAY THREE   DAY FOUR

FIVE HEALTH BENEFITS OF DRINKING WATER:

1. Brain tissue is made up of 85% water. Water helps the brain work properly.
2. Replenishing water loss during exercise is crucial for physical performance and good health. Too much water loss will increase your risk of exhaustion.
3. Thirst feels a lot like hunger. Many times, people eat instead of drink water, leading to weight gain. Drinking water fills you up and helps weight loss.
4. People who drink more than 5 glasses of water a day are less likely to die from a heart attack than people who drink less than two.
5. Drinking water flushes poisons out of the body and helps prevent pimples.

(source: sportsandcooking.com, 2008)

SODIUM MEANS SALT

- Sodium is a nutrient. It is found in salt.

- Eating too much sodium may lead to high blood pressure, which can cause strokes and other health problems.

- Sodium is used to preserve food so that it doesn't spoil and to add flavor. Canned and processed foods have large amounts of it.

- When shopping, check food labels for sodium content. You can also remove the salt shaker from the table.

- You should not have more than 2,400 mg (about a teaspoon) per day.

Match the foods on the left with the amount of sodium you think they contain.

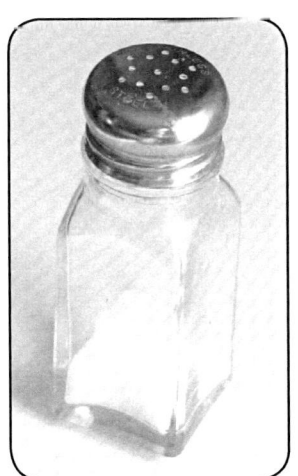

One cup of Cheerios®	2 mg.
One cup of plain oatmeal	233 mg.
One hot dog	75 mg.
A hamburger patty	875 mg.
A three-ounce can of tuna	54 mg.
Three-ounce broiled chicken breast	318 mg.

TOO MUCH SUGAR

Sugar is a major source of calories but not of vitamins and minerals. Overdosing on sweet stuff–like candy, soda, and ice cream–can make it hard to eat other foods that are healthy and loaded with vitamins.

Normally, words ending in "ose" on food and drink labels are sugars. Some examples are dextrose, fructose, glucose, maltose, lactose, and sucrose.

High fructose corn syrup is a sugar made from corn. It is cheaper to produce than cane sugar, but contains chemicals. It is the very first ingredient on this list, meaning this food item is mostly sugar and not healthy.

This food item has at least four mentions of sugar in the food label!

Dextrose is another kind of sugar. It's also known as glucose.

TOO MUCH SUGAR (CONT.)

Circle the foods that have sugar.

Mustard

Bubble Gum

Bread

Soda

Ketchup

Peanut Butter

Candy

Crackers

Pretzels

Ice Cream

Cake

French Fries

Tomato Sauce

Pancakes

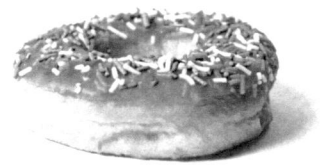

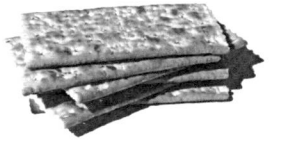

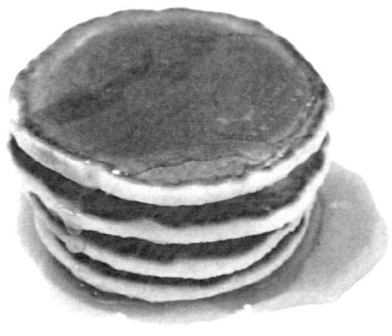

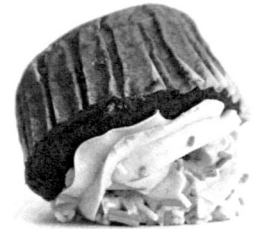

CHOICES: HEALTHY AND UNHEALTHY

Listen to your instructor's directions. Everyone is going to name foods to be listed in each column.

HEALTHY CHOICES	UNHEALTHY CHOICES

READING FOOD LABELS

A
Fruit Cup

Ingredients: peaches, water, pears, pineapple, sugar

serving size	4 1/2 ounces
servings per container	1
calories	60
carbohydrates	14 g
total fat	0 g
protein	0 g
sodium	5 mg
cholesterol	0 mg
sugar	2 mg

B
New England Clam Chowder

Ingredients: water, potatoes, clams, onions, celery, heavy cream, modified food starch, wheat flour, soy protein, onion powder, salt, yeast, sugar

serving size	1 cup
servings per container	2
calories	130
total fat	2.5 g
protein	9 g
fiber	7 g
cholesterol	5 g
sugars	0 g
sodium	480 mg

C
Fudge Brownies

Ingredients: flour, corn syrup, vegetable shortening,* sugar, water, dextrose, cocoa, eggs, walnuts, egg whites, salt, baking soda, caramel color, artificial flavors

serving size	1 brownie
calories	270
total fat	13 g
cholesterol	15 mg
sodium	170 mg
carbohydrates	40 g
fiber	1 g
sugars	28 g
protein	2 g

D
Bread

Ingredients: flour, water, corn syrup, yeast, soybean oil, salt

serving size	1 slice
servings per container	22
calories	50
total fat	1 g
cholesterol	0 mg
sodium	110 mg
fiber	1 g
sugars	1 g
protein	2 g

*This is high in saturated fat and can clog arteries in the heart.

READING FOOD LABELS (CONT.)

Use the food labels on page 49 to answer the questions below, on a per-serving basis.

1. Which food has the most calories? _____

2. How about the least calories? _____

3. The most fat? _____

4. The least fat? _____

5. Which item has the most sodium? _____

6. What about the least amount of sodium? _____

7. Which one has the most cholesterol? _____

8. What product has the least cholesterol? _____

9. List the dish that has artificial flavoring and coloring. _____

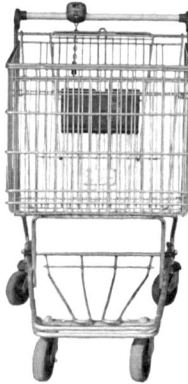

GROCERY RECEIPT

Use the following information to answer the questions on the next page.

Diet soda (2-liter)	1.50
Cereal	4.50
White bread	2.50
Salami	3.50
Bubble gum	1.00
Potato chips	3.49
Grape juice	3.75
Pineapple wedges	3.89
Swiss cheese	3.75
Corn	2.59
Steak, 10 oz.	11.00
Pop Tarts®	3.99
Rice	2.99
Potatoes	3.50
Milk	4.50
Apples (3)	2.89
Oranges (3)	<u>3.29</u>
Total	____

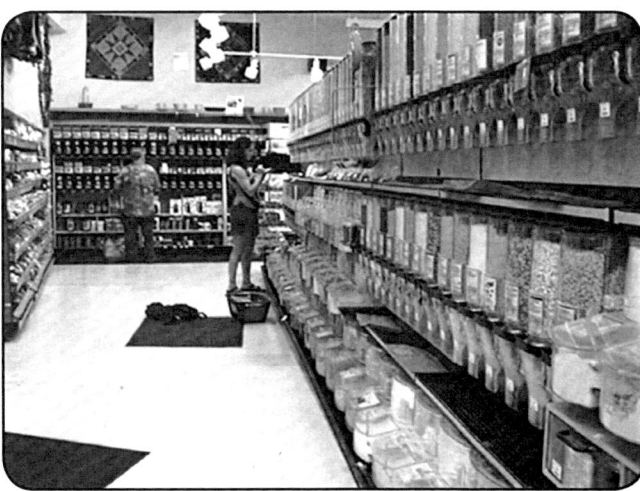

GROCERY RECEIPT (CONT.)

Use the information from page 51 to answer the following questions.

1.	Name three foods on the grocery receipt that are not healthy choices.	
2.	Now name three healthy foods on your list.	
3.	Choose three good sources of fiber. Determine their total cost.	
4.	Select three fresh food items and find how much they cost.	
5.	Which product on the list do you think has the most preservatives and chemicals?	
6.	If you only had $30, what items would you buy? Why did you choose those items?	
7.	Which items would you not buy if you wanted to eat right?	

EATING DISORDERS

1. The phrase "eating disorder" means a health-damaging eating habit that comes from psychological or social problems. People with this sickness —male or female—often overeat or don't eat at all. Their decisions about eating are based on their feelings, not on whether they're really hungry.

2. The three most common forms of eating disorders are *anorexia nervosa, bulimia,* and *compulsive overeating.* Often, these behaviors overlap, but the result is always negative. In 20 percent of anorexia nervosa cases, the result is death.

3. People with anorexia do not have a realistic body image. They always feel as if they are fat, even when they are so thin that their bodies have stopped functioning normally. Anorexics have such a fear of weight gain that they eat only very small portions of food—if they eat at all—and they may exercise too much. Women with this problem may stop having their menstrual periods or, in teenage girls, it may never begin.

4. The signs of bulimia may be less noticeable because those suffering from it usually appear to be of average weight. Bulimics go through cycles of bingeing (overeating) and purging (throwing up). During a binge, a person eats a lot of food very quickly. The person feels so uncomfortable about doing this that he gets rid of the food either by throwing up or by taking an overdose of laxatives.

5. Compulsive overeating means a person goes through periods of continuous eating. They do this in secret and cannot control it. Food is eaten to make up for feelings of loneliness or sadness, not because of hunger.

DIETING QUIZ

Place a "T" in the space before the question if the answer is true and an "F" if it is false.

1. ____ Dieting is the best way to lose weight.
2. ____ Those who diet usually have a negative image of their body.
3. ____ Dieting causes people to think about food more.
4. ____ You can eat as much as you want as long as you only eat healthy foods.
5. ____ Dieting causes people to binge on food.
6. ____ Those who diet tend to gain more weight than those who don't.
7. ____ Dieting can make you feel sad and cranky.
8. ____ You can buy healthy foods only in a health food store.
9. ____ Dieting can cause a number of physical problems.
10. ____ Dieting is all right as long as you don't eat any fats or sugars.

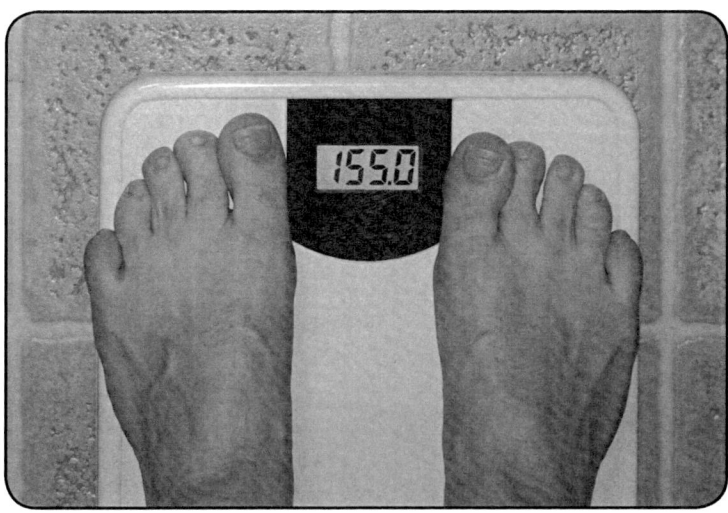

EATING PROBLEM

Write a "Y" for yes or "N" for no in the space before each question.

DO YOU...

1. ___ Starve yourself regularly?
2. ___ Overeat and then make yourself vomit?
3. ___ Feel out of control when you sit down to have a meal?
4. ___ Feel a sense of power and control when you don't have any food?
5. ___ Binge on food when you are having negative feelings?
6. ___ Feel you do not deserve to have food?
7. ___ Know the calorie count in each of the items you eat?
8. ___ Feel the only control you have is over food and your weight?
9. ___ Believe you are fat — even when people say you're not?
10. ___ Feel you have to do everything perfectly?
11. ___ Use laxatives or diet pills to control your weight?
12. ___ Exercise to burn calories instead of to stay fit?
13. ___ Keep secrets about your eating habits?
14. ___ Get angry at anyone who asks questions about your eating habits?
15. ___ Feel guilty after a big meal?
16. ___ Believe that you're ugly and worthless?
17. ___ Not go to parties because there might be chips and dip?
18. ___ Think about food all the time?
19. ___ Believe that life will be perfect if you lose weight?
20. ___ Fear gaining weight?
21. ___ Think that you may have an eating disorder?

WHAT I THINK OF MY BODY

List all the good, positive thoughts you have about your body in the left column. Then, in the right column, write down all the negative thoughts you have about your body. Finally, cross off the list on the right and remember no one is perfect. Even with your pimples and scars, you are still a beautiful human being.

POSITIVES	**NEGATIVES**
_____	_____
_____	_____
_____	_____
_____	_____
_____	_____
_____	_____
_____	_____
_____	
_____	

DANGER SIGNS

Read each of the situations below and put an "X" in the box beside the people you think show signs of an eating disorder. Write which type you think each one is. If you think the person doesn't have an eating disorder, write "none." Use the information on worksheet page 53, Learner's Workbook page 20 to help you.

SITUATION	DANGER	POSSIBLE DISORDER?
Julie is in the eighth grade and of average height and weight, but she feels she's too fat. Every day, she has only vegetables and exercises for at least one hour.		
Although overweight, Jack goes home after school and inhales a grilled cheese sandwich and French fries. It makes him feel better because he is lonely. Even though he feels guilty after eating, he can't stop.		
Samantha looks good, but she doesn't feel that way. Some days, she eats so much that she feels sick to her stomach. But she thinks she's okay because she takes laxatives or makes herself throw up, and therefore hasn't gained any weight.		
Sheila is conscious of her weight, so she stays away from sweets and exercises three times a week. She feels good about herself and is happy with her body.		

ATTITUDE CHANGES

Read each sentence out loud. What do you think about these statements? Do you agree or not?

- I realize that being thin or having bulging muscles does not make me a better person.

- Always feeling tired and drinking too much coffee and soda in an effort to jumpstart my body isn't such a good idea.

- I realize that changing negative eating habits isn't easy, but I'm going to work on it.

- I'm going to be aware of what I say about people's bodies and how my comments make that other person feel.

- I'm going to boost my immune system by eating healthy.

- I understand that TV and magazines don't always show realistic bodies, so I'm going to like me more.

- I can cut my health risks from overeating, undereating, drinking, and smoking by changing how I feel about these habits. From now on, I will block diseases by living and eating smart.

> "Our attitude toward life determines life's attitude toward us."
> —*John N. Mitchell*

UNDERSTANDING MYPLATE

MyPlate illustrates the five food groups that are the building blocks for a healthy diet. . Before you eat think of what goes on your plate, select a food group below.

MyPlate says make half of your plate fruits and vegetables. MyPlate is based on the 2010 Dietary Guidelines for Americans.

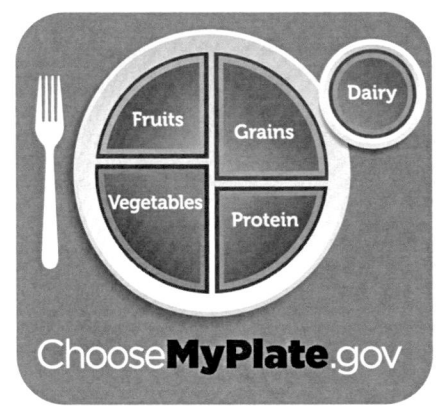

1. **Fruits:** Any fruit or 100% fruit juice is part of the fruit group/ Fruits may be fresh, canned, frozen, dried, and maybe put whole, cut or pureed.

2. **Vegetables:** Any vegetable or 100% vegetable juice is part of the vegetable group. Vegetables may be raw, cooled, fresh, frozen, canned and may be whole, cut-up, or mashed. Based on their nutrient content, vegetables are organized into 5 subgroups: dark green vegetables, starch vegetables, red and orange vegetables, beans and peas.

3. **Grains:** A food made from wheat, rice, oats, cornmeal, barley or another cereal grain is a grain product. Bread, pasta, oatmeal, breakfast cereals, tortillas, and grits are examples of grain products. Grains can be whole grains. Examples of whole grains are whole wheat flour, brown rice, oatmeal, whole cornmeal. Grains can be refined. These have been milled and have the bran and germ removed. This gives grains a finer texture and improves their shelf life, but it also removes dietary fiber, iron and many B vitamins. Some examples of whole grains are white flour, white bread and white rice.

4. **Protein Foods:** All foods made from meat, poultry, seafood, beans and peas, eggs, processed soy products, nuts, ad seeds are considered part of the protein group. Select a variety of protein foods to improve nutrient intake and health benefits, including at least 8 ounces of cooked seafood per week. Young children need less, depending on their age. Vegetarians get their protein from beans and peas, nuts and seeds. Meat and poultry should be lean or low-fat.

5. **Dairy:** All milk products are part of this group. Diary choices should be fat-free or low-fat. Foods made from milk that retain their calcium content are part of this group. Foods made from milk that have little to no calcium, such as cream cheese, cream, and butter, are not. Calcium fortified soy milk is part of the diary group.

UNDERSTANDING MYPLATE (CONT.)

The biggest group is the pasta, grains, bread, and cereal group. We should eat six servings of these foods daily. This means cereal at breakfast, bread for lunch (whole grain is best), rice or pasta for dinner, plus snacks from this group. A slice of bread equals one serving.

Moving through the plate, the next groups are fruits and vegetables. We should eat three to five servings of fresh vegetables a day and two to four servings of fruit. Canned fruits and vegetables are okay, but fresh fruits and vegetables are better. One cup of raw vegetables or a half cup of fruit juice equals one serving.

The dairy group—milk, yogurt, and cheese—should be eaten two to three times per day; however, many dairy products are high in fat, so it is important to read labels and buy low-fat items. One cup of milk equals one serving.

Meat, poultry (chicken and turkey), fish, dried beans, eggs, and nuts are high in protein. We need two to three servings of these a day. One serving means two to three ounces (about two thin slices of turkey).

Not included in the plate are foods we should not eat too much of: fats, oils, and sweets. These include candy, cakes, soda, cookies, ice cream, and other junk food. Fats make us fat and can cause heart trouble. Sugar causes
cavities and can make us jittery. Too much salt can cause high blood pressure.

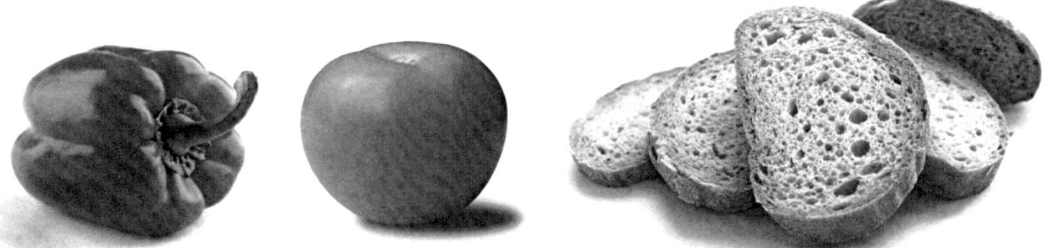

A RACE AGAINST TIME

On the lines below, write one healthy food beginning with each letter. For these purposes, don't worry about grammar and spelling. Just do the best you can. The main idea is for you to participate.

A_____   N_____
B_____   O_____
C_____   P_____
D_____   Q_____
E_____   R_____
F_____   S_____
G_____   T_____
H_____   U_____
I_____   V_____
J_____   W_____
K_____   X_____
L_____   Y_____
M_____   Z_____

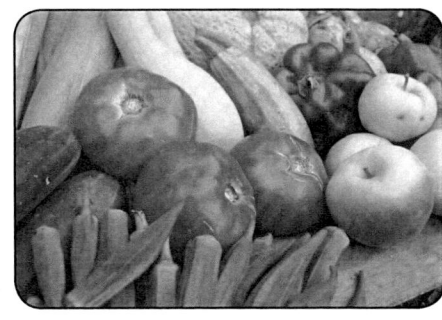

THE BLANK MYPLATE

Fill in the plate below with examples of foods from each category. Be as creative as you want. Not all of us are born artists. Just do the best you can.

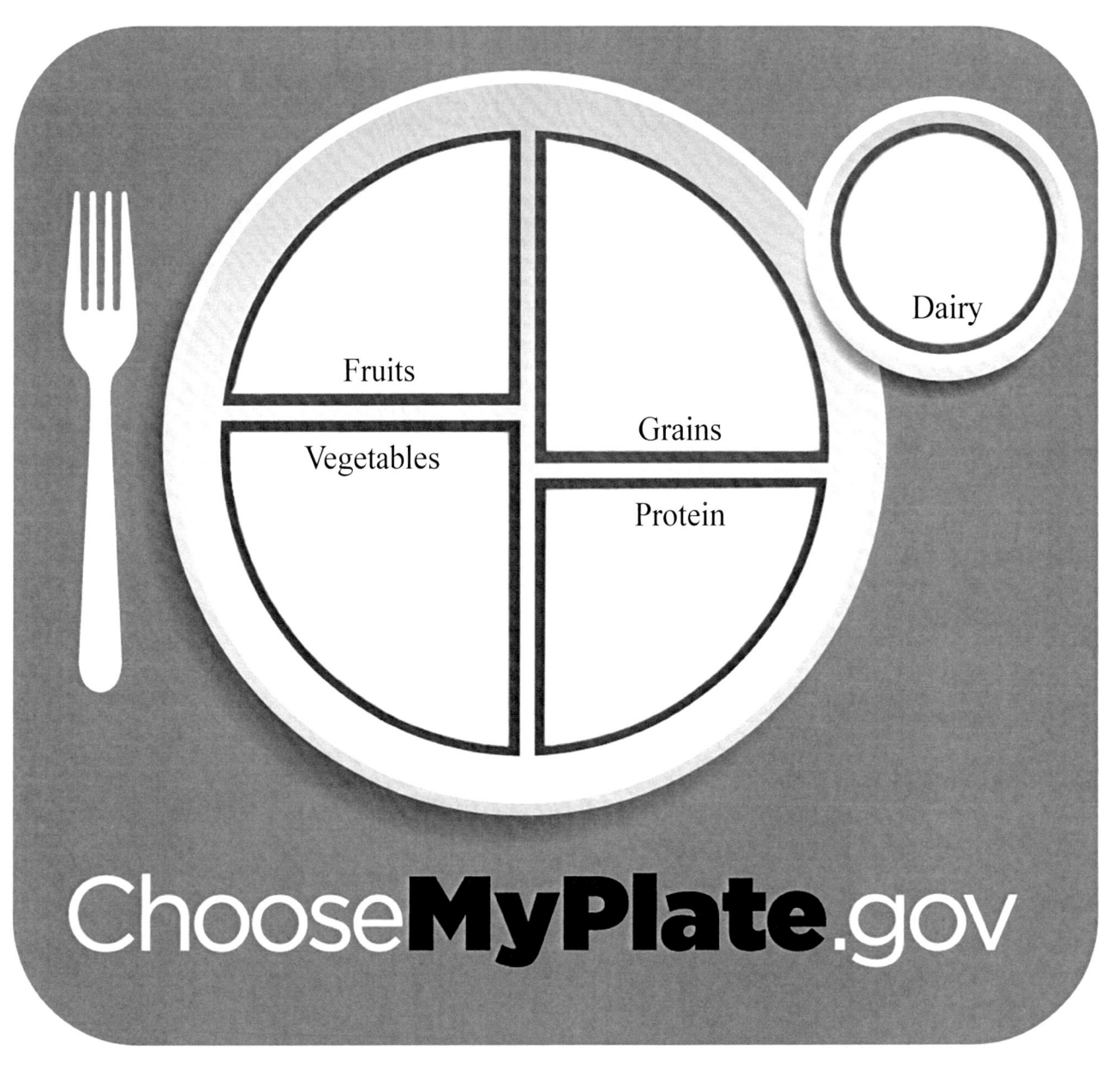

Planning Meals

Design two menus: one with healthy meal choices, and the other with unhealthy meal choices.

BREAKFAST

HEALTHY CHOICE

LESS HEALTHY CHOICE

LUNCH

HEALTHY CHOICE

LESS HEALTHY CHOICE

DINNER

HEALTHY CHOICE

LESS HEALTHY CHOICE

MAKING CHANGES

Write down what you usually eat every day. Then, decide if you have a healthy diet or if you need to make changes. For these purposes, don't worry about grammar and spelling. Just do the best you can.

WHAT I USUALLY EAT	CHANGES I WILL MAKE
BREAKFAST	
LUNCH	
DINNER	
SNACKS	

FAVORITE FOODS

List your favorite foods under each heading. Are you making healthy food choices? For these purposes, don't worry about grammar and spelling. Just do the best you can. The main idea is for you to participate.

FRUITS AND VEGETABLES	MEATS
DAIRY	PASTA, GRAINS, BREADS

TYPES OF NUTRIENTS

Using the word bank at the bottom of this page, fill in the FOOD EXAMPLES column.

FOOD EXAMPLES

PROTEIN	
CARBOHYDRATES	
VITAMINS	
MINERALS	
FATS	
FIBER	

WORD BANK

meat	potatoes	A, B, C, D, E
fish	iron	breads
mayonnaise	whole grains	vegetables
calcium	butter	chicken

SEARCH FOR PROTEIN

Find and circle all the protein-rich foods listed in the word bank. Answers may be across, down, backward, or diagonal.

```
F I S H B A H G R A I N S F
A L E A U A A N I T M I L K
M O A A C G C D M U R E M V
I R T A K R L L D R T C N E
C E M A E A K E J K A H B G
S H N A T I N S H E T E M E
T A I A S N N A K Y A E P T
E T V C E S A W L I R S O A
A A A S K A E N P P A E D B
K G C F G E R U F R T Y C L
B E A N S L N T N E R S A E
E G G S F R I S E M E A T S
```

Word Bank

meat	chicken	turkey	fish
milk	cheese	eggs	grains
beans	nuts	vegetables	steak

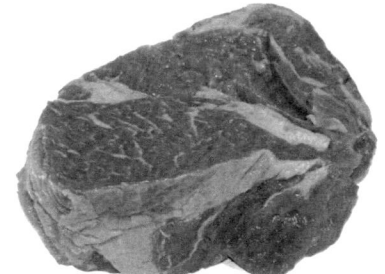

CHEER FOR PROTEIN

Read the following paragraph and then write a short summary that convinces someone to eat the proper amount of protein. For these purposes, don't worry about grammar and spelling. Just do the best you can. The main idea is for you to participate.

> Protein repairs damaged body cells and builds new muscle and tissue. Foods high in protein include meat, poultry, fish, dairy products, and eggs. The average American eats four times more protein than he needs. Most of it comes from hamburgers, ribs, steak, ham, pork chops, chicken, turkey, and cheese. While some protein every day is important in our diet, people end up eating too much. Some proteins are high in fat. Remember, fats are the smallest part of MyPlace. Eat proteins that are lowest in fat (fish, lean meats, egg whites, beans and nuts).

_____

_____

_____

_____

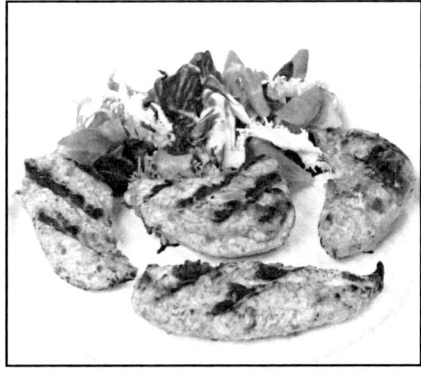 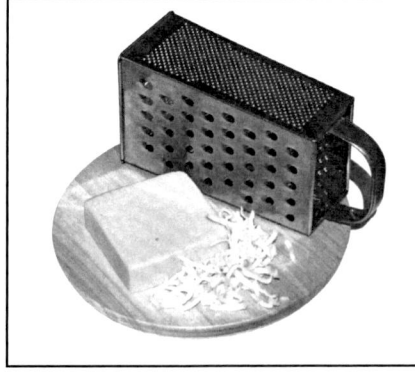 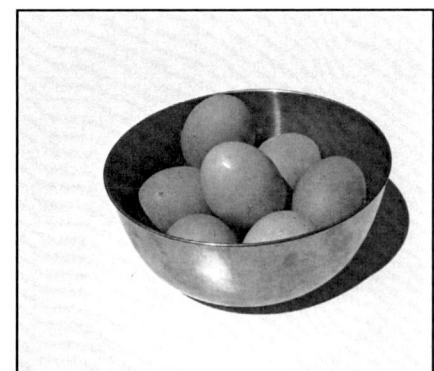

ALL ABOUT CARBOHYDRATES

Read the information in each shape out loud.

Carbohydrates are energy foods. They are converted into glucose (sugar) and used by the nervous system, muscles, and liver. Carbohydrates don't give you long-term energy, though. If you eat of a lot of them at once, you have a lot of energy at first, but "crash" later.

Simple sugars are used by the body quickly. Whatever you don't burn off with exercise is converted to fat. Foods like chocolate, cookies and cake are loaded with so much simple sugar that most of it is converted to fat.

Complex grains provide energy and nutrients the body needs. Complex grains are healthier than simple sugars, but still need to be limited, because whatever you don't burn off with exercise is converted into fat.

Fiber helps us digest food. Some high-fiber foods are asparagus, carrots, squash and broccoli.

Starch is found in all carbohydrates. A few examples of starchy foods are brown rice, potatoes, kidney beans, lima beans and bread.

CARBO FUEL

Circle the foods high in complex carbohydrates. Put an X through foods high in simple carbohydrates (sugar).

Soda

Fruit drinks

Candy

Whole-wheat bread

Cookies

Cheerios®

Bagel

Pastry

Lemon drops

Pretzel

Chewing gum

Baked potato

Fruit Loops® cereal

Oatmeal

Doughnut

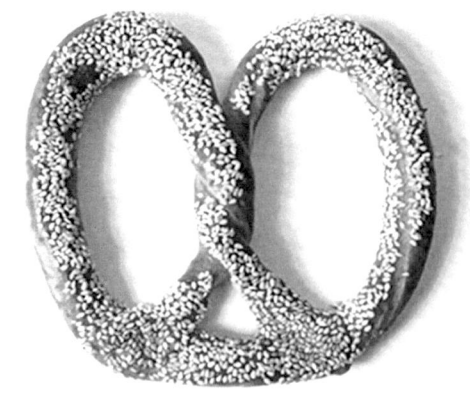

THUMBS UP/THUMBS DOWN

In the "thumbs-up" column, list carbohydrates that are good for you. In the other one, list those that are not as healthy. You should try to eat more complex carbohydrates and less simple carbohydrates. For these purposes, don't worry about grammar and spelling. Just do the best you can. The main idea is for you to participate.

Complex Carbohydrate	**Simple Carbohydrate**

ALL ABOUT FIBER

We should try to eat 20 to 30 grams of fiber a day. Use the chart below to add up all the foods you would need to equal 20 grams of fiber. Put a check mark next to those items.

	FOOD	AMOUNT	FIBER (GRAMS)
☐	Kidney beans	1/2 cup	7
☐	Pinto beans	1/2 cup	6
☐	Lima beans	1/2 cup	4
☐	Banana	1 medium	4
☐	Dried figs	3	4.6
☐	Strawberries	1/2 cup	3
☐	Carrots, raw	1 cup	3
☐	Whole-wheat bread	1 slice	2
☐	Baked potato with skin	1 medium	4
☐	Brown rice	1 cup	4
☐	Apple	1 medium	3
☐	Hot dog	1 medium	0
☐	Chicken	1 piece	0
☐	Wheat flakes	1 oz.	2.5
☐	White bread	1 slice	0.5

VITAMIN WEB

Fill in the information below. In each large oval, write down what that vitamin does for the body; in the outer circles, list foods that contain it. (Vitamin A has been done as an example.) For these purposes, don't worry about grammar and spelling. Just do the best you can. The main idea is for you to participate.

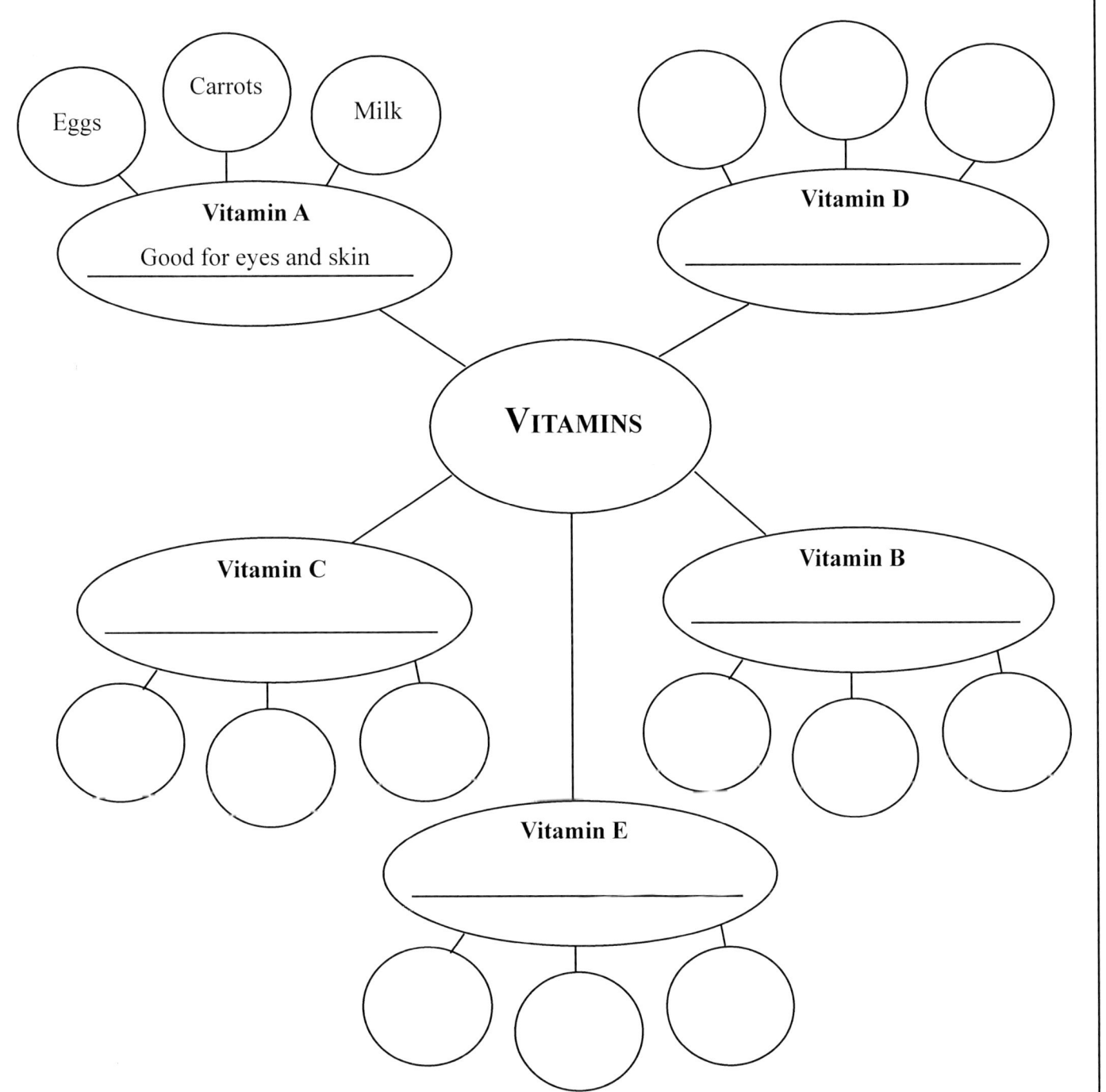

ARISE Basic Health 101: Nutrition and Exercise, Instructor's Manual, Page 73

Vitamins and Minerals In Your Diet

Read the paragraph below and use that information to write the correct vitamin- or mineral-rich food in each box.

Many foods have vitamins built right in. If you eat enough of the proper ones, you will not need to take pills. Citrus fruit, such as oranges and grapefruit, is full of vitamin C, which helps fight off colds. Some vegetables, such as broccoli, have a lot of iron. This makes our blood cells work properly. Beta-carotene from carrots keeps our eyes healthy. Calcium from cheese and vitamin D from milk strengthen our bones and teeth.

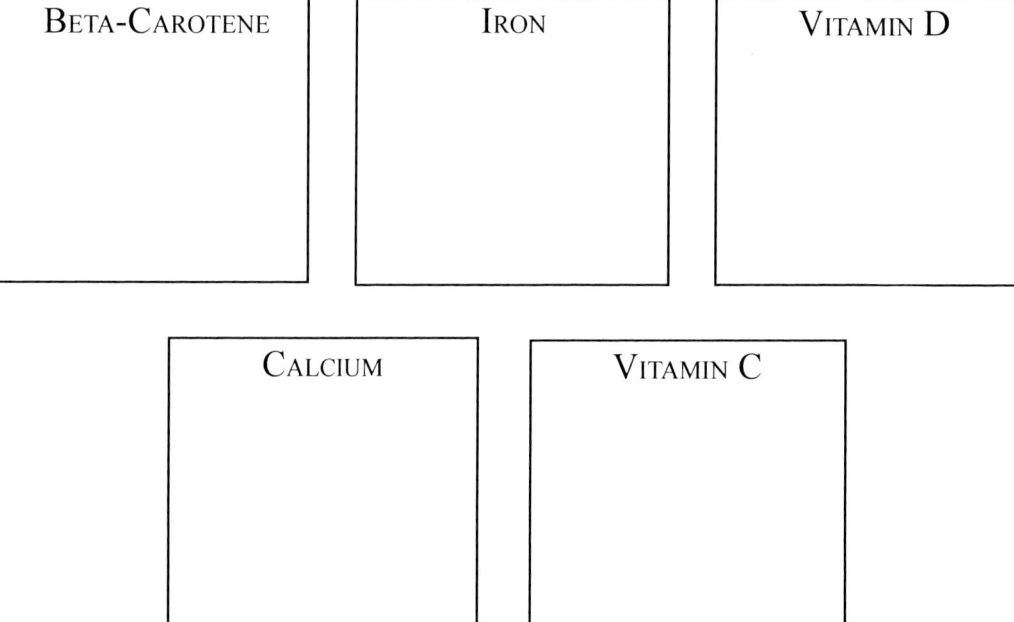

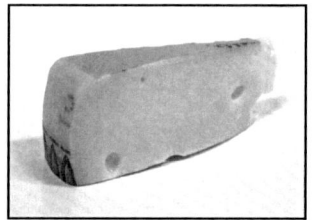 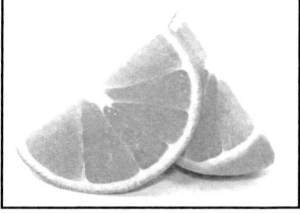 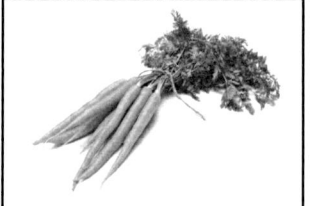 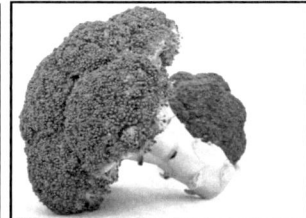

Minerals

```
         MINERALS
         /      \
    CALCIUM    IRON
```

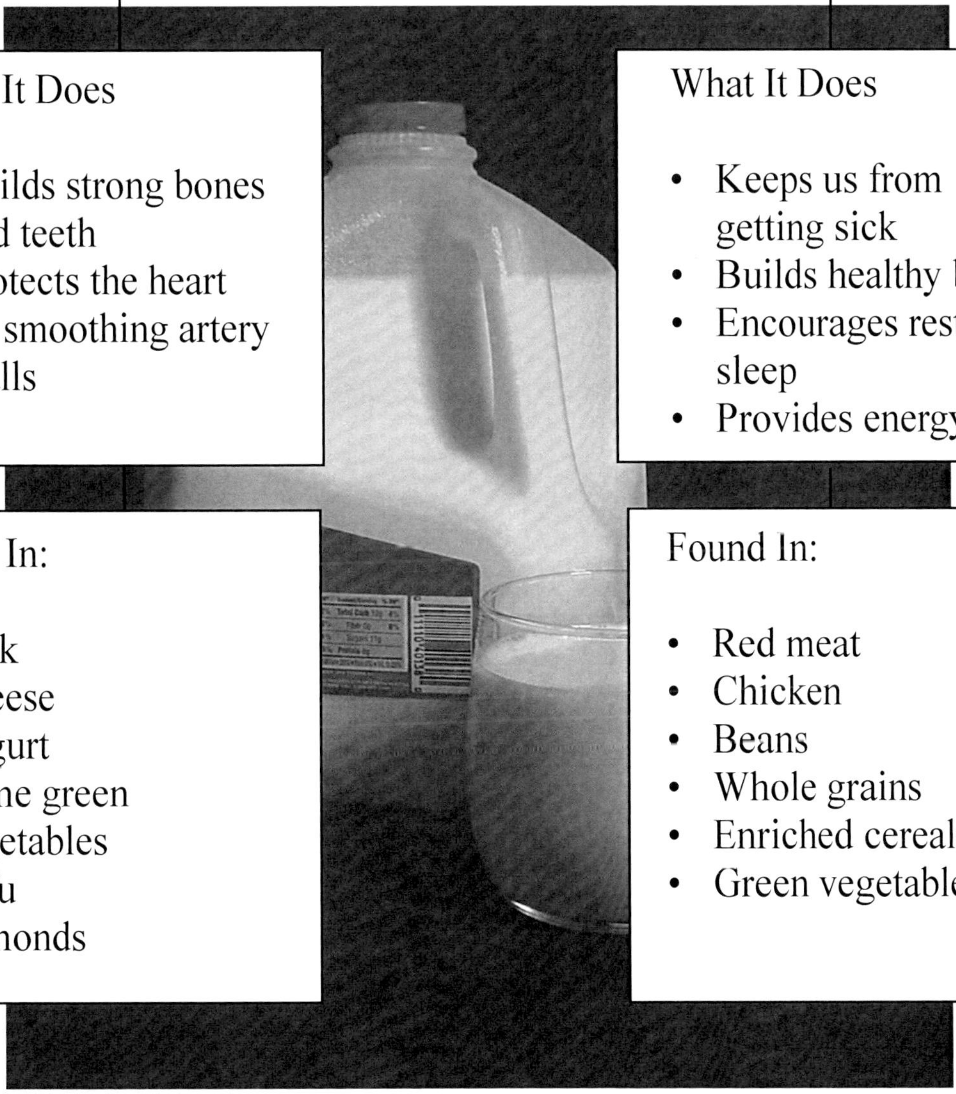

What It Does

- Builds strong bones and teeth
- Protects the heart by smoothing artery walls

Found In:

- Milk
- Cheese
- Yogurt
- Some green vegetables
- Tofu
- Almonds

What It Does

- Keeps us from getting sick
- Builds healthy blood
- Encourages restful sleep
- Provides energy

Found In:

- Red meat
- Chicken
- Beans
- Whole grains
- Enriched cereals
- Green vegetables

Restaurant Menus and Minerals

Choose foods from each of the menus that are high in iron and calcium. Circle your choices.

Menu 1
Appetizers: mozzarella sticks, pizza breadsticks, stuffed mushrooms, yogurt, fruit

Salads: mixed greens, chicken Caesar, spinach and tomato

Entrees: lasagna, spaghetti, plain pizza, chicken and vegetable pizza

Vegetables: broccoli, carrots, corn

Dessert: low-fat yogurt, chocolate cake

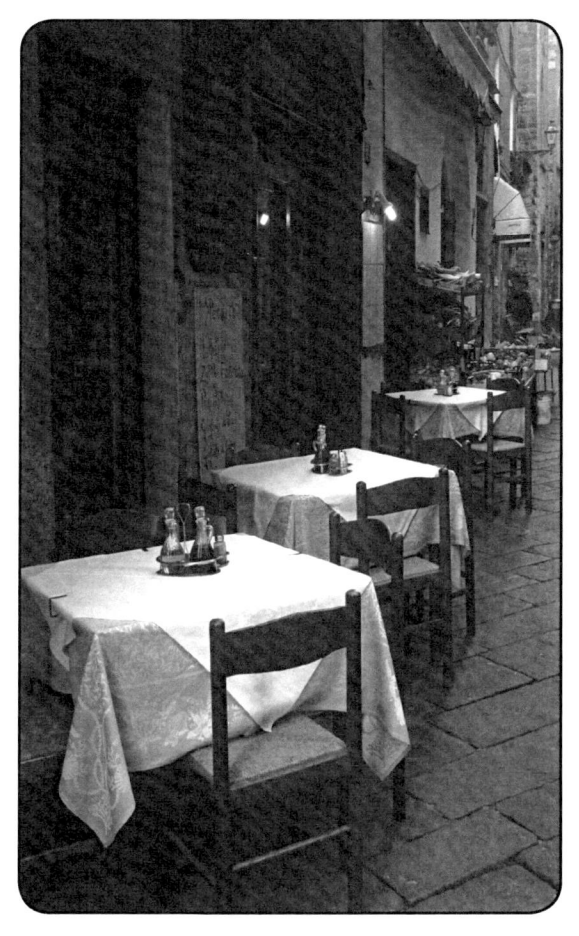

Menu 2
Appetizers: shrimp cocktail, cottage cheese with fruit

Salads: leafy greens with tomato and onion, bean salad

Entrees: chicken parmesan, shrimp with tomatoes and peppers, meatloaf, steak

Vegetables: creamed spinach, red beans and white rice, lima beans and yellow rice

Desserts: strawberries topped with low-fat whipped cream, chocolate pudding

Facts About Fat

Read the paragraph below, then answer the questions by writing a "T" for true or an "F" for false on the line before each statement.

Fat is a nutrient our body needs. We use it for energy, body heat and maintaining healthy body tissues. Fat can be divided into three groups: polyunsaturated *(pah-lee-uhn-sat-chur-a-ted)*, monounsaturated, and saturated. Unsaturated fats are necessary, but saturated fats (found in butter, bacon, cheese, and cookies) clog the arteries and veins just like grease stops up a sink's drain. They increase our risk of getting heart disease and strokes. Fast food is frequently high in both fat and salt, so be sure to make wise choices when eating at those restaurants. Choose plain hamburgers, baked potatoes, and salads. Avoid dressings, sour cream, cheese, and mayonnaise; these are high in fat. Use lemon juice instead of salad dressing—it's a very friendly food!

_____ 1. Unsaturated fats are unhealthy.

_____ 2. Foods high in saturated fats increase the risk of heart disease.

_____ 3. Fast foods are generally not high in fat.

_____ 4. You cannot eat healthy at a fast-food restaurant.

_____ 5. It's necessary to eat some fats.

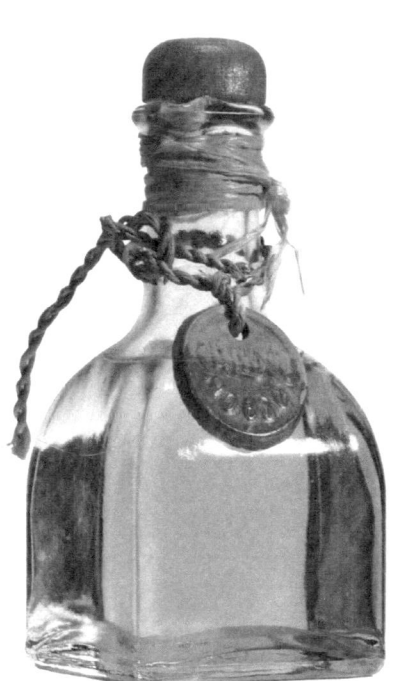

ARISE Basic Health 101: Nutrition and Exercise, Instructor's Manual, Page 77

FAT MAKES FAT COMIC STRIP

Create a food character—like a talking banana in a supermarket—who points out which products are smart healthy foods and those that are not, and turn it into a comic strip. Not all of us are born great artists. Do the best you can to satisfy yourself.

- Read labels and look for hidden fats.
- Look at the food; if it is greasy, it is loaded with fat.
- All oils are fats.
- All dairy foods have fats (unless the label says "fat free").
- All fried foods are high in fat.
- Always choose low-fat foods over fatty foods.

Defining Physical Fitness

Physical fitness is the overall condition of a person's body.

Health-related fitness refers to the best levels of flexibility, cardiorespiratory endurance (the ability of the heart, lungs, and circulatory system to provide nutrients during activities), muscular strength, and body composition (how much fat and muscle you have).

Sports-related fitness includes the elements of health-related fitness, but focuses on coordination, agility, reaction time, and speed. Sports-related fitness is limited by what the body can do; for example, training does little to improve reaction time.

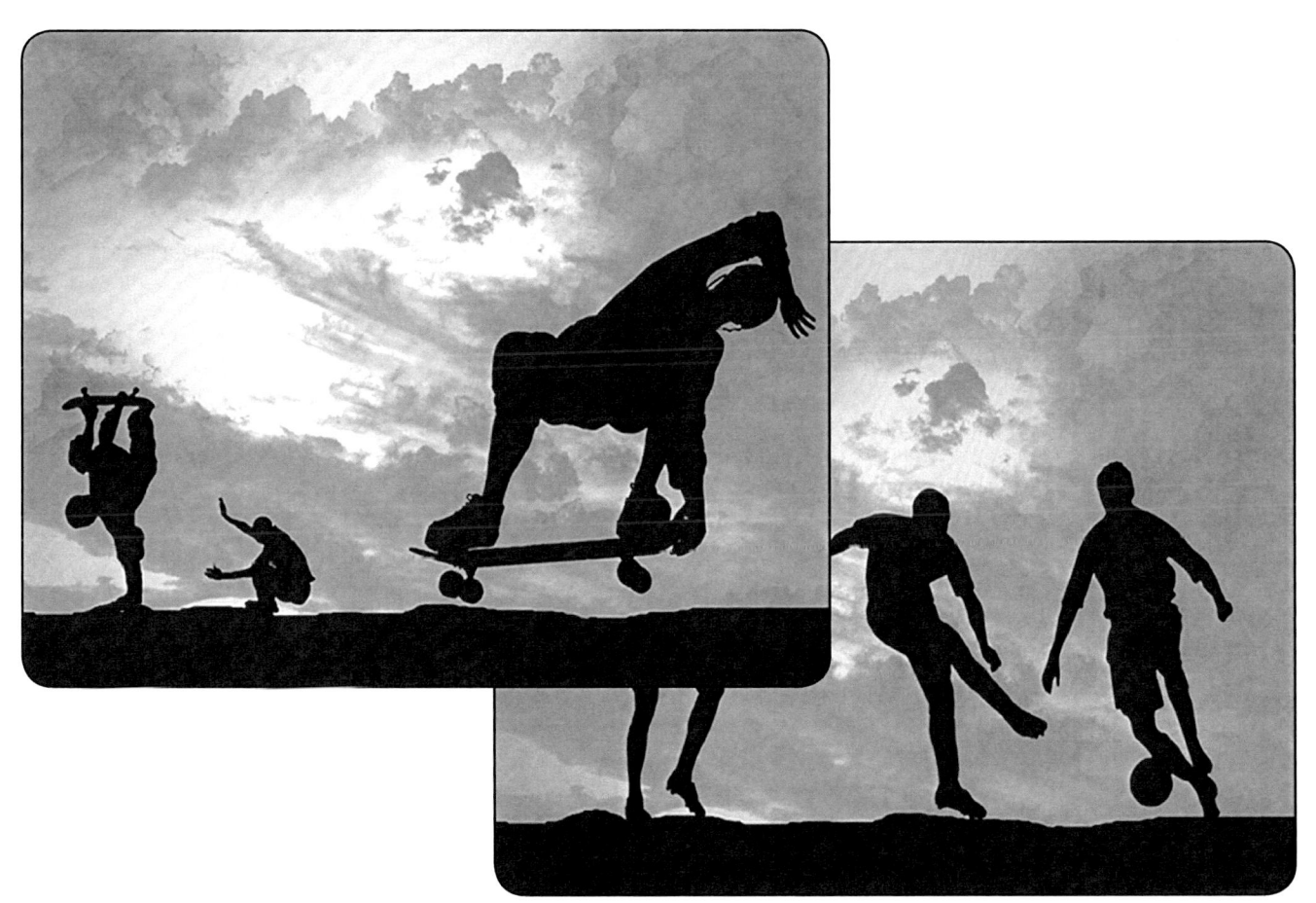

MY OWN PHYSICAL FITNESS

Write about your favorite physical activity. For these purposes, don't worry about grammar and spelling. Just do the best you can. The main idea is for you to participate.

_____
_____
_____
_____
_____
_____
_____
_____
_____
_____
_____

COMPONENTS OF PHYSICAL FITNESS

Put a check mark next to the items that are health-related, sports-related, or both. If it doesn't apply to either one, mark it with a zero.

COMPONENT	HEALTH RELATED	SPORTS RELATED
Cardiorespiratory endurance (ability of the heart and lungs to work for long periods of time)		
Flexibility (ability to move your joints through a full range of motion)		
Muscular strength (how much force your muscles can take)		
Agility (ability to change position or direction quickly)		
Muscular endurance (ability to use your muscles for a long period of time)		
Reaction time (the time it takes you to move after realizing the need to act)		
Body composition (levels of lean muscle and fat in your body)		
Speed (ability to cover distance in a short amount of time)		
Balance (ability to maintain posture while standing or moving)		

CARDIOVASCULAR FITNESS: IN YOUR OWN WORDS

1. Cardiovascular fitness (the ability of the heart, lungs, and circulatory system to provide muscles with oxygen) is one of the most important factors in total fitness.

2. People who have cardiovascular fitness feel better, have less body fat, and are able to stay active for longer periods of time.

3. Cardiovascular fitness reduces the risk of heart disease.

4. Aerobic exercise increases the heart rate and provides an excellent cardiovascular workout.

5. Aerobic exercise includes fast walking, jogging, cycling, rollerblading, jumping rope, swimming and much more.

6. Pay attention to the intensity (how hard), duration (length), and frequency (how often) of your exercise. This all determines cardiovascular fitness.

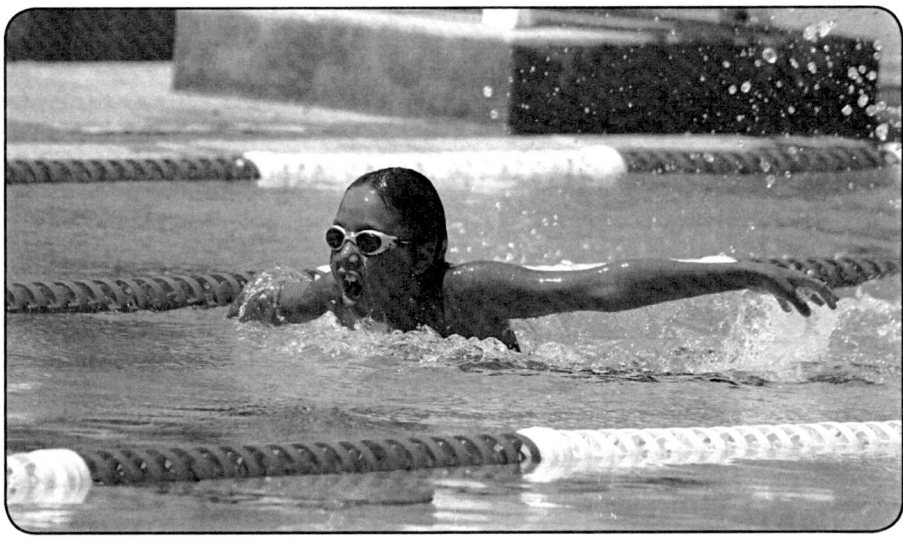

DESIGN AN EXERCISE ROUTINE

Imagine you are a coach of a sports team that is going to play a championship on Saturday. Starting on Monday morning, design a week's worth of exercises for your athletes. For these purposes, don't worry about grammar and spelling. Just do the best you can. The main idea is for you to participate.

_____
_____
_____
_____
_____
_____
_____
_____
_____
_____
_____
_____
_____
_____

FACTS AND BENEFITS: TRUE OR FALSE QUIZ

Write a "T" for true or "F" for false on the line before each statement.

_____ 1. Exercise can help your skeletal structure (your bones).

_____ 2. Exercise can help your heart work better.

_____ 3. Exercise causes a temporary rise in blood pressure.

_____ 4. Exercise can make the arteries (the pathways that pump blood to the rest of your body) in your heart healthier.

_____ 5. Exercise can make your lungs stronger.

_____ 6. The best exercise is the hardest one you can do.

_____ 7. Exercise can help your brain.

_____ 8. Exercise can lower your blood cholesterol level.

_____ 9. You burn calories and fat only when you are exercising.

_____ 10. Running is a type of aerobic exercise.

EXERCISE IS GOOD FOR EVERYTHING

Read the health benefits of regular exercise below. Then, write a letter to a friend explaining why it's important to exercise. For these purposes, don't worry about grammar and spelling. Just do the best you can. The main idea is for you to participate.

- ☐ Your resting heart rate is lower because your blood pressure goes down and the heart does not have to work as hard to get blood to your body.
- ☐ The heart is better able to send blood where it is needed in the body.
- ☐ Your blood can carry more oxygen.
- ☐ Arteries become healthier.
- ☐ Blood cholesterol decreases.
- ☐ You make less adrenaline *(ah-dren-ah-lihn)* in response to emotional stress.
- ☐ Exercise reduces tension and related headaches and improves sleep.
- ☐ It also heightens creativity, sharpens concentration, and improves decision-making abilities.

Dear _____ ,

_____

_____

_____

_____

_____

_____

Sincerely,

_____

Ways To Exercise

There are many ways to exercise. Write about the different types and what part of the body they affect. What type of equipment do you need? What are the rules? For these purposes, don't worry about grammar and spelling. Just do the best you can. The main idea is for you to participate.

_____
_____
_____
_____
_____
_____
_____
_____

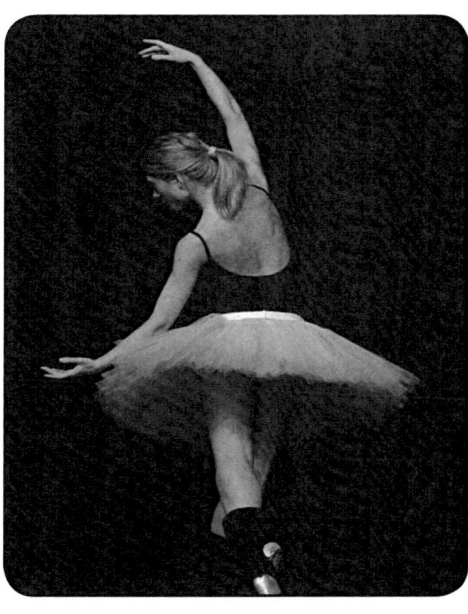
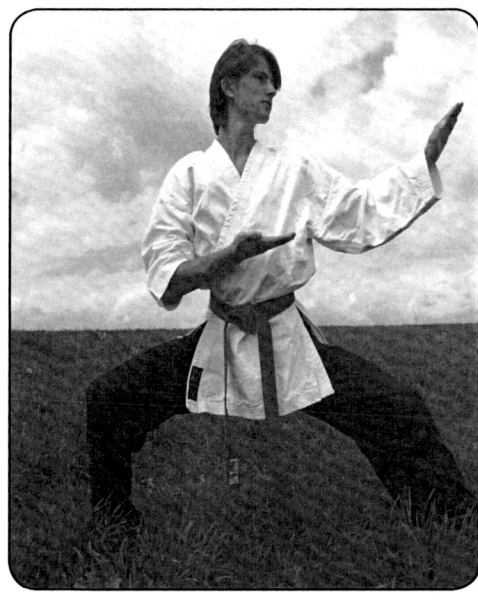

WALKING MAP

Read the following tips. Then, draw a map of your neighborhood showing places you can walk to as part of your daily exercise.

- ☐ Choose a time of day that works for you. Write down the hour you will start. Don't be late!

- ☐ If you're not in shape, start with a short stroll; 10 to 15 minutes is a great beginning. Then, gradually increase your speed and how long you stay out.

- ☐ Wear comfortable shoes and clothing suitable for the weather. This means no sweatpants when the temperature outside is 90 degrees.

- ☐ Walk in a natural way—heel to toe—and allow your arms to swing naturally. Breathing deeply also helps.

- ☐ Cool down by going more slowly toward the end of each session. Don't sprint on your way home and then suddenly stop. Ease into it.

THE PLEDGE TO EXERCISE

I, _____ (name), pledge to make exercise a part of my daily life because it will make me healthy and strong. It also helps my mental well-being.

I pledge to try to get my family involved in daily workouts as well.

I understand that there are many ways that I can make it fun and not just another chore like taking out the garbage.

For instance:
- ❐ I can go for a short walk after dinner each night.
- ❐ I can schedule exercise with a friend two or three times a week.
- ❐ I can go for walks on Monday and play ball on Saturday.
- ❐ I can take the stairs instead of the elevator.
- ❐ I can ride a bike for short distances instead of driving or taking a bus.

Here are three more ways I can make working out a daily part of my life:

_____

_____

_____

Signed this _____ day of _____, 20 _____

_____
(Your signature)

DEFINING FLEXIBILITY

Flexibility, a health-related part of physical fitness, is the ability to move the body through a full range of motion.

- It allows us to function at our best and lets us move freely without stiffness, muscle soreness, or injury.

- Stretching is the only way to improve flexibility.

- Exercises, such as neck bends, calf and wall stretches, are great for the joints and ligaments (large, tough tissues that connect your bones).

- All these activities must be done *slowly* to avoid injury.

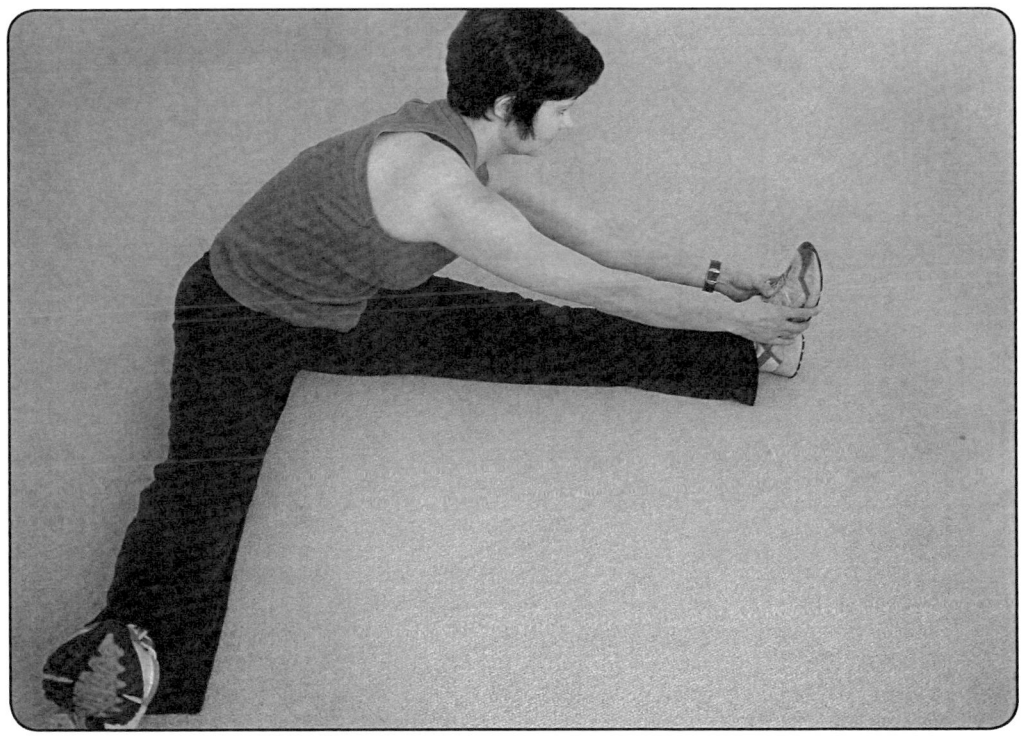

WORKING AT FLEXIBILITY

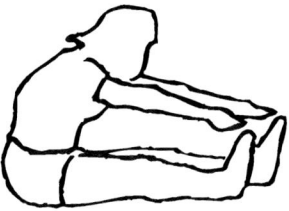

Sit and reach (low back and hamstring stretch)

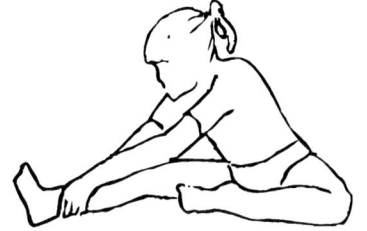

Hurdler's stretch

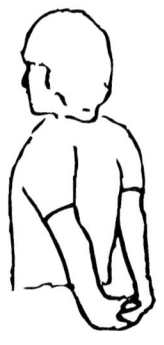

Shoulder and pectoral stretch

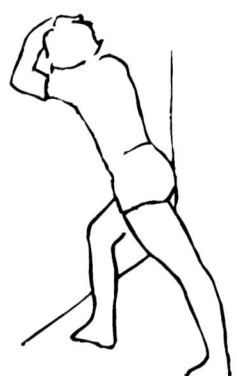

Wall stretch (calf and Achilles stretch)

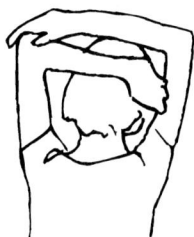

Upper back and shoulder stretch

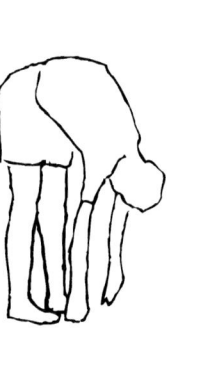 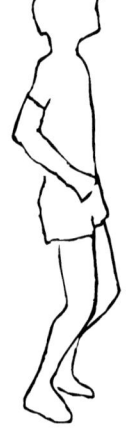 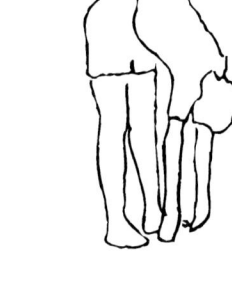

Touch toes

Working at Flexibility (cont.)

Yoga Stretching Exercises

We have found these exercises to be wonderful in keeping limber and feeling tip top. As you work your way through, affirm that every day in every way that you're better and better.

Use moderation move ahead step by step. Eliminate any exercise that causes discomfort particularly in you lower back area.

Starting Posture:

Stand erect
Feet together
Palms together
Relax

Inhale
Feel the clean
fresh air nourishing
your body.

Exhale
Stale old air
from your systems
and release tension

Position 1

Lean back as far as is comfortable.

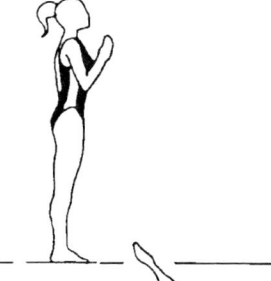

One deep inhalation.

Position 2

Increase your position slowly, carefully, in your day-by-day step-by-step.

Don't try to get this far down all at once! Do the best that you can.

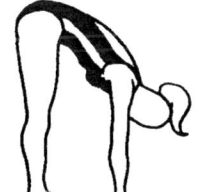

One deep inhalation.

Position 3

Right foot back.

Head up — **gently**

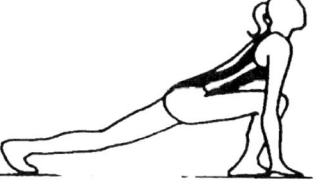

One deep inhalation.

Use gentle consistency

WORKING AT FLEXIBILITY (CONT.)

Position 4

Keep you body straight.

Visualize a more supple you.

Be gentle.

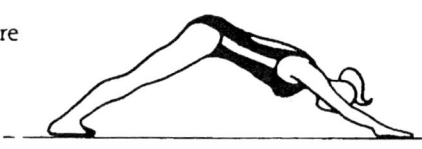

As you exercise, feel clean fresh air nourishing your system. Stale old air exiting your body releasing all tension. You feel great.

Position 5

Lower your body to the floor —slowly try to match this position: hands, chest, knees, toes on the floor.

Next lower the entire body in preparation for next postion.

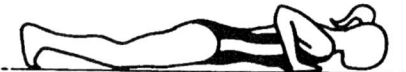

One exhalation.

Position 6

Lift chest and midsection gently.

Slowly, develop this position Remember to visualize a more beautiful limber you.

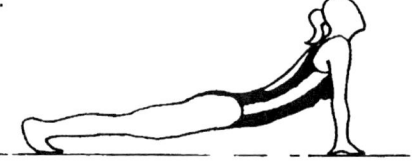

Deep inhalation.

Position 7

Place your body in this position

Your goal is to eventually have your feet flat on the floor.

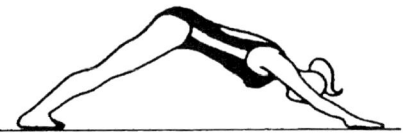

Exhalation.

Moderation

WORKING AT FLEXIBILITY (CONT.)

Position 8

Bring right foot to the level of hands.

Look up.

Work slowly and diligently into this position

This is the same as Position 3 only that the right foot instead of the left is in the between-hands position

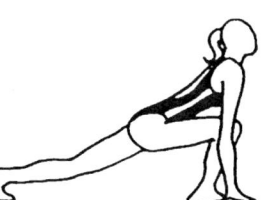

As you exercise, feel clean fresh air nourishing your system. Stale old air exiting your body releasing all tension. You feel great.

Inhalation.

Position 9

Bring left leg forward at the same time the body is bent matching the position in 2.

Easy does it.

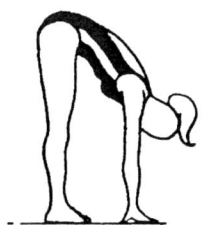

Exhalation.

Position 10

Raise arms as you did in Position 1

Bend backward gently. Stay within your realm of competency, but work very slowly toward a maximum!

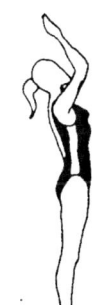

Inhalation.

Closing Poture:

Same as the starting posture.

Feel the energy —it's almost as if your body is thanking you for this workout.

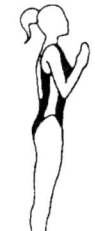

Exhalation and ordinary breathing.

Be Gentle Time Is On Your Side

FLEXIBILITY TRAINING PRINCIPLES

Use these guidelines to develop a healthy stretching workout.

Frequency: At least three times per week; gradually increase the number of sessions per week or per day.

Intensity: Stretch slowly until you feel mild tension in your muscles. Each time, try to increase the distance stretched.

Time: Stretch for 15 to 30 seconds. Perform more repetitions with each routine.

Type: Do a slow, steady stretch. Don't bounce!

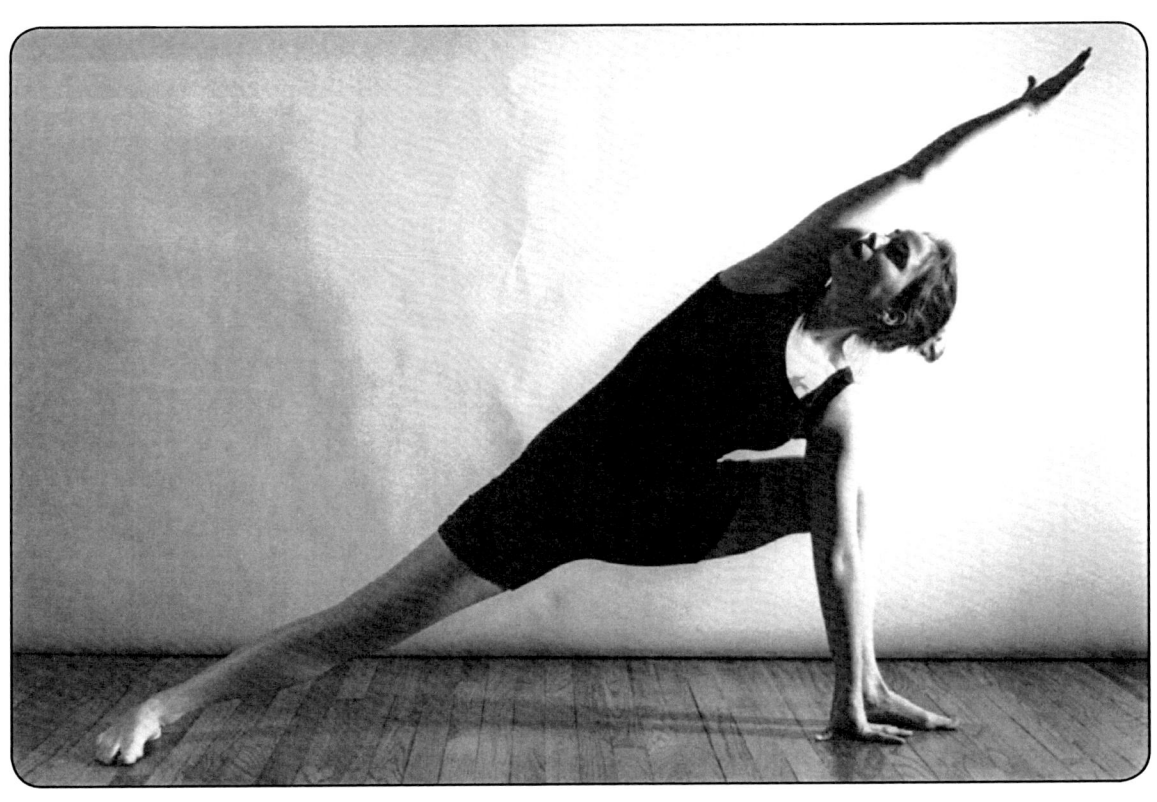

Source: Adapted from *Personal Fitness and You*, North Carolina Hunter Textbooks (1993).

DEFINING MUSCULAR STRENGTH

Muscular strength is the amount of force a muscle can exert. It contributes to good health and proper body functions. Without this, we would be unable to perform our best at work or play.

Muscular strength can be improved in many ways. For a muscle to become strong, it must work harder than it did before.

There are two kinds of muscle-building exercises: **isometric** and **isotonic**.

Isometric exercises contract (squeeze) the muscles when pushing against an object or another body part; examples include push-ups and pressing your arms against a door frame.

Isotonic activities involve contracting the muscles while moving a resistance, such as barbells or hand weights. Weightlifting is an isotonic exercise.

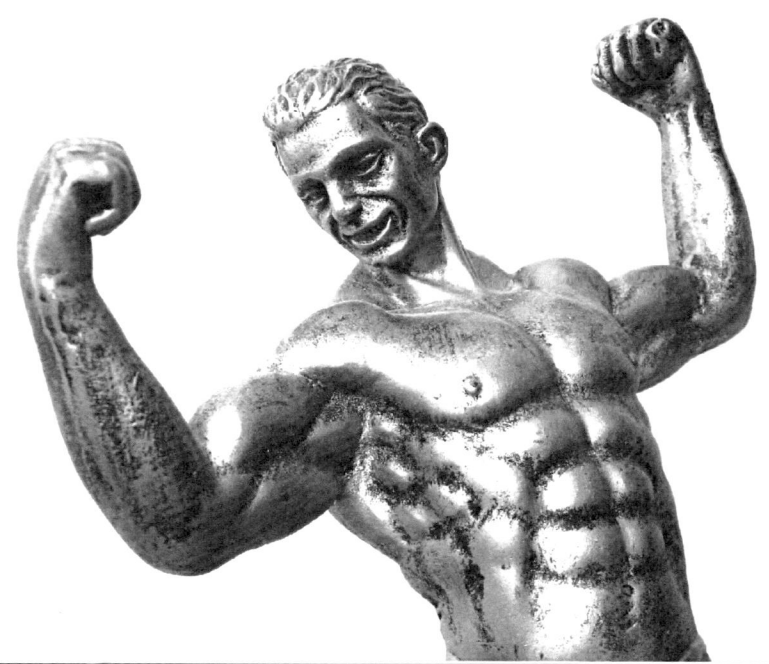

Muscular Strength Word Find

Find and circle the words in the word bank. Answers can be horizontal, vertical, or diagonal.

```
W I S O M E T R I C M A N I T O N
E A N S A Y O S T O J B O A F E A
I O S T R E A M Y S F Y B D U X A
G M I R E S I S T A N C E C N E B
H O W U S N L K U R S I S I A R P
T E F R E Q S E L T E J R U C C O
T U O A K E J I O S C A M K T I W
R N I M T I O S T E U E D N A S E
A F R E Q U E N C Y W C A M J E R
I M A G K S A E T A T Y M O I L A
N L C D U R A T I O N H U C A L O
I S O T O N I C R T D A C W P K L
N R D G U E T O M U S C L E J M U
G S O L C R H Y U I A G U P A G Y
B A R E N D U R A N C E T E C L O
```

Word Bank

intensity	resistance	duration	endurance	isometric	power
treadmill	exercise	isotonic	frequency	muscle	weight training

ACTIVITY LOG

List all the physical activities that you do in an average day.

7 a.m. _____
8 a.m. _____
9 a.m. _____
10 a.m. _____
11 a.m. _____
Noon _____
1 p.m. _____
2 p.m. _____
3 p.m. _____
4 p.m. _____
5 p.m. _____
6 p.m. _____
7 p.m. _____
8 p.m. _____
9 p.m. _____
10 p.m. _____
Other: _____

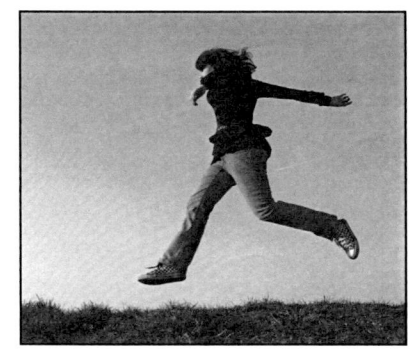
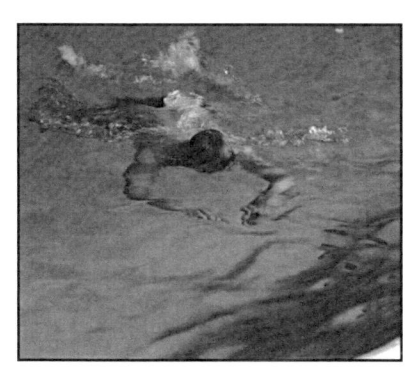
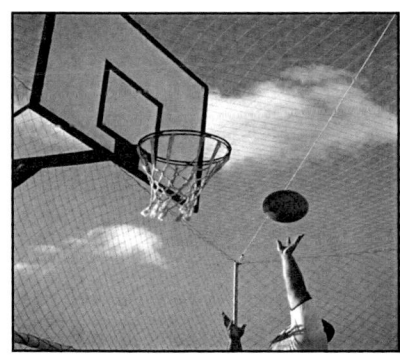

ARISE Basic Health 101: Nutrition and Exercise, Instructor's Manual, Page 97

VOCABULARY

Adrenaline *(uh-dren-uh-lin)*: chemical produced by the body that helps us exercise and deal with stress.

Agility *(uh-jil-i-tee)*: ability to change position or direction quickly.

Anorexia nervosa *(an-or-ex-ee-uh nur-vo-suh)*: unrealistic fear of weight gain that causes the sufferer to starve himself.

Arteries *(ar-tuh-rees)*: the tubes your heart pumps blood through.

Ballistic stretching *(bah-lis-tik)*: uses a lot of bouncing; can cause rips and tears in delicate tissue surrounding the joints (knee, elbow, etc.) if not done correctly.

Beta-carotene *(bay-tuh kar-uh-teen)*: substance found in red, orange, yellow, and dark green vegetables that is changed into vitamin A by the body.

Body composition *(com-po-zi-shun)*: levels of muscle and fat in the body.

Bulimia *(bul-i-mee-uh)*: constant craving for food, often marked by bingeing (eating large amounts of food) and purging (vomiting).

Calcium *(kal-see-um)*: a mineral needed in the diet to build strong bones and teeth.

Carbohydrate *(kar-bo-hy-drayt)*: sugars and starches.

Cardiorespiratory endurance *(kar-dee-oh-res-pir-tor-ee)*: ability of the heart and lungs to work for long periods of time.

Cardiovascular fitness *(kar-dee-oh-vas-kyu-lar)*: ability of the heart, lungs, and circulatory system to provide oxygen that muscles need.

Cholesterol *(co-les-ter-awl)*: a soft, waxy, fat-like substance used in the body.

Compulsive *(cum-pul-siv)*: when you can't stop yourself from doing something.

Diabetes *(dy-uh-bee-teez)*: disease in which urine and blood contain excess sugar.

Duration *(dur-ay-shun)*: length of time.

Fatigue *(fah-teeg)*: tiredness.

Fiber *(fy-bur)*: vegetable substances that are digested partially or not at all.

Flexibility *(flex-uh-bi-li-tee)*: ability to move the body through a full range of motion.

Frequency *(free-kwen-see)*: how often you do something.

Vocabulary (cont.)

Grains *(grayns)*: seeds or fruits of some food plants like wheat or oats.

Intensity *(in-ten-si-tee)*: an amount of force needed to do something.

Isometric *(i-so-met-rik)*: muscle-building exercises which contract (squeeze) the muscles when working against an object or other body part; for example, push-ups.

Isotonic *(i-so-ton-ik)*: muscle-building exercises which contract muscles while moving a resistance such as weights; for example, weightlifting.

Laxative *(lax-uh-tiv)*: a drug that relieves constipation (being unable to have a bowel movement) and sometimes used by those with eating disorders.

Menstrual *(men-stru-al)*: having to do with a female's monthly period.

Mineral *(min-ur-al)*: a chemical element in the earth and human bodies that is neither animal nor vegetable, needed for growth and many body functions.

Nutrients *(nu-tree-ents)*: substances that promote growth.

Nutritionist *(nu-trish-uh-nist)*: a person who teaches people how to eat healthy.

Nutritious *(nu-trish-us)*: healthy.

Osteoporosis *(ahs-tee-o-por-o-sis)*: disease in which bones are weak and easily broken.

Protein *(pro-teen)*: nutrient found in meat, fish, chicken, turkey, and nuts, needed by the body for growth and cell repair.

Psychological *(sy-ko-lah-ji-kal)*: relating to the science of the mind and behavior.

Saturated fat *(sah-tyur-ay-ted fat)*: usually solid at refrigerator temperature, this fat raises blood cholesterol levels; found in meat, poultry, dairy, and tropical oils.

Sodium *(so-dee-um)*: salt.

Stationary stretching *(stay-shun-air-ee)*: moving the joints of the body slowly to their maximum range.

Unsaturated fat *(un-sah-tyur-ay-ted fat)*: type of fat that stays liquid at refrigerator temperature; there are two types: polyunsaturated (safflower, sunflower, and soybean oils) and monounsaturated (olive and canola oils).

Vitamins *(vi-ta-menz)*: substances needed by the body in tiny amounts, found in food.

ARISE Basic Health 101: Nutrition and Exercise

Worksheet Answers

www.ariselife-skills.org

Review Activity Crossword Worksheet: *Page 25*

Across
2. vitamins
3. eating disorder
5. fats
6. mineral
8. sodium
10. bones

Down
1. fiber
4. grains
7. pyramid
9. legumes

A Balanced Diet Word Search Worksheet: *Page 38* **Learner's Workbook:** *Page 5*

```
D X J U E E I N I S T I U R F
F L X V G B Q C H Q C N O P S
G C Y G O V O O H E A L T H Y
P Z H Z C Y N Y A D R W E R U S
S K K S N F S H U I W N C Y N
N N M Y I S E L B A T E G E V
R F I B A F T D E Y N R F V H
I O E A E E O L E Y N G U E F
O R D E I R R L K Y M Y H M B
T F N A R G P I L T Z M Z D V
Y R T V L R W V K F Y C F T X
I E O E G W R C J D D Q J X
D A P X M F L D U Z W E M Q
```

What Do You Know? Food Categories Worksheet: *Page 39* **Learner's Workbook:** *Page 6*

1. Carbohydrate 2. Iron, Calcium, Vitamin C 3. Vitamin A, Iron, Vitamin C, Calcium, Fiber 4. Calcium, Protein, Vitamin A 5. Calcium, Protein, Vitamin A 6. Protein, Fats/Oils, Vitamin E 7. Carbohydrate, Fiber, Vitamin C 8. Protein 9. Fiber, Protein, Iron 10. Vitamin C, Fiber 11. Iron, Protein 12. Fiber, Vitamin C

What Do You Know? Food Facts Survey Worksheet: *Page 40* **Learner's Workbook:** *Page 7*

1. True
2. True
3. True
4. True
5. True
6. True
7. False
8. True
9. False *(Explanation:* Vitamin pills are vitamin *supplements.* This means they are a way of getting the vitamins your body needs when you are not getting enough of them from the foods you eat. It's cheaper and better for your body to eat the right foods instead of spending money on vitamins.)
10. True

NUTRITION AND EXERCISE WORKSHEET ANSWERS (CONT.)

Nutritional I.Q. Quiz Worksheet: *Page 41*　　　　**Learner's Workbook:** *Page 8*
1.　　**d. 10 teaspoons.** Drinking a bottle of soda is like drinking artificially flavored seltzer water with 10 teaspoons of sugar dissolved in it. In fact, soda is the largest single source of sugar in the American diet. We get 10 times more sugar from sodas than we do from candy.
2.　　**a. The cheeseburger** packs more than seven times as much sodium as the French fries. Even the apple pie contains four times as much sodium as the fries and the milk shake twice as much! The French fries just taste saltier because the salt is on the surface. People who are trying to cut back on sodium should realize that high-sodium processed foods don't always taste salty. The salt is mixed with other ingredients and is swallowed before you can taste it.
3.　　**b. The Triple Cheeseburger** is truly a "Heart Attack Special." The cheesecake is not a low-fat food but, at 240 calories (of which 60 percent is fat), it is healthier than the cheeseburger. The Wendy's creation has 1,040 calories, with about the same percentage of fat as the dessert.
4.　　**b. True.** A medium apple has four grams of fiber.

Benefits of Healthy Foods Worksheet: *Page 42*　　**Learner's Workbook:** *Page 9*
beans, sugar, emotions, mental, overeating, American, natural, memory, appetite, brain

Sodium Means Salt Worksheet: *Page 45*　　**Learner's Workbook:** *Page 12*
One cup of Cheerios = 233 mg of sodium
One cup of plain oatmeal = 2 mg of sodium
One hot dog = 875 mg of sodium
A hamburger patty = 75 mg of sodium
A three-ounce can of tuna = 318 mg of sodium
Three ounces broiled chicken breast = 54 mg of sodium

Reading Food Labels Worksheet: *Pages 49-50*　　**Learner's Workbook:** *Pages 16-17*
1. C　　2. D　　3. C　　4. A　　5. B　　6. A　　7. C　　8. A or D　　9. C

Grocery Receipt Worksheet: *Pages 51-52*　　**Learner's Workbook:** *Pages 18-19*
grocery receipt total: $62.63
1. potato chips, Pop Tarts®, bubble gum, salami
2. pineapple wedges, Swiss cheese, corn, rice, potatoes, milk, apples, oranges
3. cereal, apples, oranges, potatoes, cost varies depending on which three
4. pineapple wedges, potatoes, apples, oranges, cost varies depending on which three
5. potato chips, Pop Tarts®, salami
6. answers can vary based on learners' opinions
7. diet soda, white bread, salami, bubble gum, potato chips, Pop Tarts®, 10-oz. steak

NUTRITION AND EXERCISE WORKSHEET ANSWERS (CONT.)

Dieting Quiz Worksheet: *Page 54*   **Learner's Workbook:** *Page 21*
1. F (The best way to lose weight is to eat a healthy diet and have sweets and fats only in moderation.)
2. T
3. T
4. F (Too much of any food can be bad for you.)
5. T
6. T
7. T
8. F (Healthy foods can be bought in regular stores also; often more cheaply.)
9. T (Constipation, headaches, and dizziness are a few of them.)
10. F (Dieting is not all right. The best way to lose weight is to eat a healthy balanced diet.)

Danger Signs Worksheet: *Page 57*   **Learner's Workbook:** *Page 24*
Julie: X, Anorexia Nervosa; Jack: X, compulsive overeating; Samantha: X, bulimia; Sheila: No X, none

Types of Nutrients Worksheet: *Page 66*   **Learner's Workbook:** *Page 33*
Proteins: meat, fish, chicken; Carbohydrates: potatoes, vegetables, whole grains, bread; Vitamins: A-E; Minerals: calcium, iron; Fats: mayonnaise, butter; Fiber: whole grains, vegetables, potatoes.

Search For Protein Worksheet: *Page 67*   **Learner's Workbook:** *Page 34*

F	I	S	H	B	A	H	G	R	A	I	N	S	F
A	L	E	A	U	A	N	I	T	M	I	L	K
M	O	A	A	C	G	C	D	M	U	R	E	M	V
I	R	T	A	K	R	L	L	D	R	T	C	N	E
C	E	M	A	E	A	K	E	J	K	A	H	B	G
S	H	N	A	T	I	N	S	H	E	T	E	M	E
T	A	I	A	S	N	N	A	K	Y	A	E	P	T
E	T	V	C	E	S	A	W	L	I	R	S	O	A
A	A	A	S	K	A	E	N	P	P	A	E	D	B
K	G	C	F	G	E	R	U	F	R	T	Y	C	L
B	E	A	N	S	L	N	T	N	E	R	S	A	E
E	G	G	S	F	R	I	S	E	M	E	A	T	S

NUTRITION AND EXERCISE WORKSHEET ANSWERS (CONT.)

Carbo Fuel Worksheet: *Page 70*   **Learner's Workbook:** *Page 37*
Learners should circle pretzels, whole-wheat bread, baked potato, Cheerios, oatmeal, bagel; and put an "X" on everything else.

Vitamin Web Worksheet: *Page 73*   **Learner's Workbook:** *Page 40*
Vitamin A is good for the eyes and skin. It is found in carrots, eggs, milk, yellow and orange fruits and vegetables, and other foods.
Vitamin B comes in several forms, is good for the nerves and helps the body use carbohydrates, fats, and protein for energy. It is found in peanuts, meats, cereals, whole grain breads, and in some vegetables and fruits.
Vitamin C helps build strong bones and teeth, heal cuts and burns, and keep the body strong. Vitamin C is found in citrus fruits (oranges, lemons, limes, grapefruits), berries, and green vegetables.
Vitamin D is called the "sunshine vitamin" because our bodies produce it when our skin receives sunlight. It is found in milk and cheese and helps make our bones and teeth strong.
Vitamin E protects our cells from damage and may help prevent cancer. It is found in green vegetables, vegetable oils, nuts, seeds, whole grain breads, cereals, and wheat.

Facts About Fat Worksheet: *Page 77*   **Learner's Workbook:** *Page 44*
1. F   2. T   3. F   4. F   5. T

Facts and Benefits: True or False Quiz Worksheet: *Page 84*   **Learner's Workbook:** *Page 51*
1. True
2. True
3. True
(*Explanation:* Although your heart rate and blood pressure will rise while you are exercising, your resting heart rate and blood pressure will decrease—a sign of a healthier body.)
4. True
5. True
6. False
(*Explanation:* Vigorous exercise, such as running, bicycling, speed skating, and team sports, are effective. However, walking regularly, swimming, or bicycling at your own pace or stretching on a regular basis are good ways to begin to maintain a healthy lifestyle.)
7. True
8. True
9. False
(*Explanation:* Regular exercise raises your metabolism, so even when not exercising, you will burn calories and fat faster than someone who never exercises.)
10. True

Nutrition and Exercise Worksheet Answers (cont.)

Muscular Strength Word Find Worksheet: *Page 96*   **Learner's Workbook:** *Page 63*

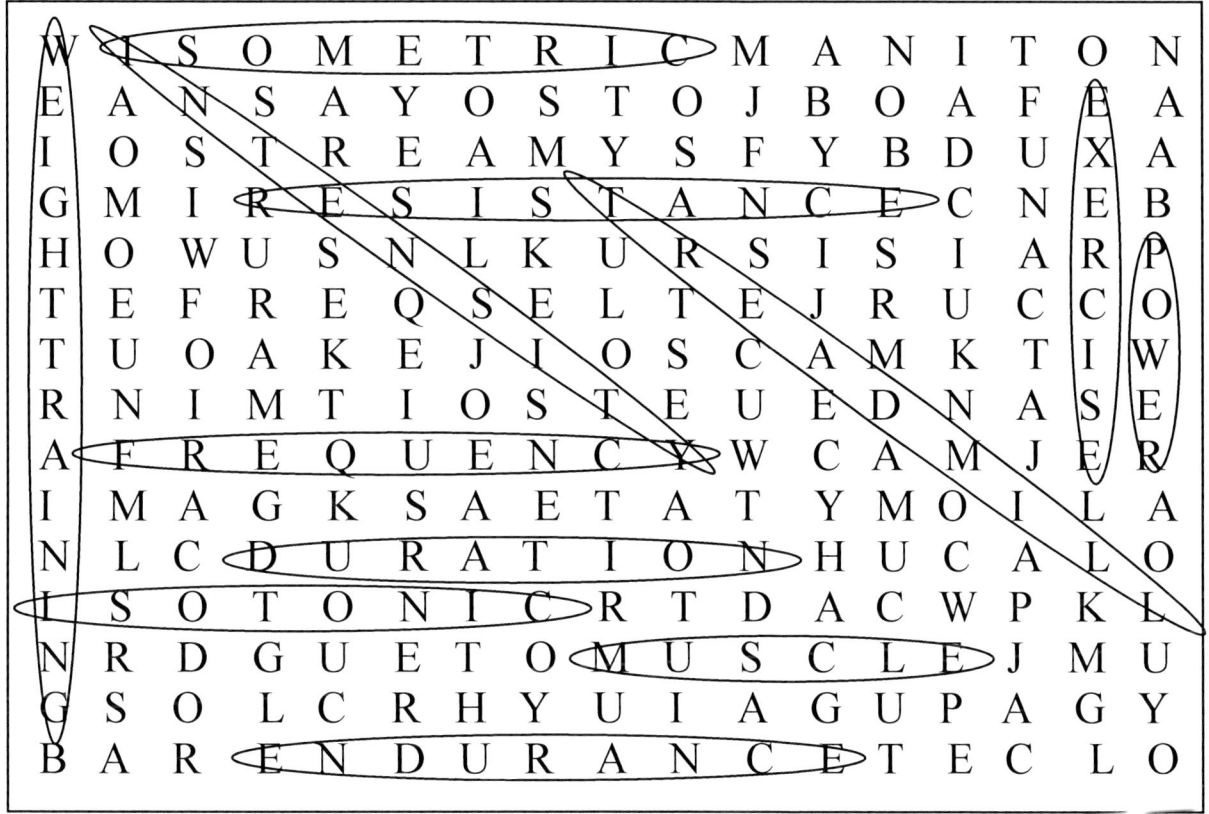

ARISE Basic Health 101: Nutrition and Exercise, Instructor's Manual, Page 105

ARISE Basic Health 101: Health and Hygiene

Quizzes and Assessments

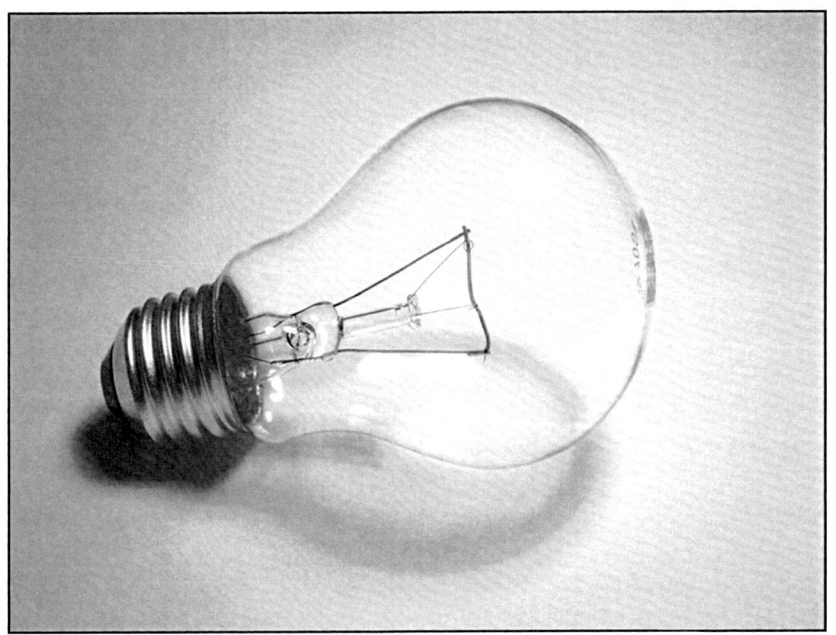

www.ariselife-skills.org

NUTRITION AND EXERCISE
SECTION 1 QUIZ

Name: _____   Date: _____

Circle the correct answer for each statement.

1. A good diet contains:
   - a. a lot of fat
   - b. a little fat
   - c. no fat
   - d. none of the above

2. Which of the following has fat?
   - a. potato chips
   - b. cake
   - c. oil
   - d. all of the above

3. Food labels will tell you:
   - a. if a food tastes good
   - b. how a food fits into your daily diet
   - c. how much fat, sodium, cholesterol, and protein the food contains
   - d. both b and c are correct

4. Food labels can be found on most _____ of food and beverages.
   - a. boxes
   - b. cans
   - c. bottles
   - d. all of the above

5. Eating healthy food can:
   - a. improve your body image
   - b. prevent you from getting sick
   - c. improve your state of mind
   - d. all of the above

NUTRITION AND EXERCISE
SECTION 2 QUIZ

Name: _____   Date: _____

Circle the correct answer for each statement.

1. MyPlace is:
   a. a guide to eating well
   b. a sandwich
   c. found in Egypt
   d. none of the above

2. You should eat _____ to _____ servings a day from the pasta, grains, and bread group.
   a. two to five
   b. six
   c. five to seven
   d. none of the above

3. Not counting fats, oils, and sweets, there are ____ basic food groups.
   a. four
   b. six
   c. five
   d. none of the above

4. Potatoes are a:
   a. carbohydrate
   b. fat
   c. protein
   d. mineral

5. Which food has the most fiber per serving?
   a. whole-wheat bread
   b. kidney beans
   c. baked potato
   d. both a and c are correct

NUTRITION AND EXERCISE
SECTION 3 QUIZ

Name: _____   Date: _____

Circle the correct answer for each statement.

1. Body composition refers to:
   a. amount of force your muscles can exert
   b. the amount of fat in your body
   c. the ability to move parts of your body through a full range of motion
   d. none of the above

2. A stretch should be held for _____ to _____ seconds to be effective.
   a. five to 10
   b. 15 to 30
   c. 10 to 20
   d. none of the above

3. Frequency refers to how _____ you should exercise:
   a. hard
   b. fast
   c. often
   d. none of the above

4. Which of the following is not a kind of muscle exercise?
   a. isotetric
   b. isotonic
   c. isometric
   d. none of the above

5. Aerobic exercises include:
   a. jogging
   b. rollerblading
   c. cycling
   d. all of the above

NUTRITION AND EXERCISE ASSESSMENT

Name: _____   Date: _____

TRUE/FALSE

Write a "T" for true or "F" for false on the line before each statement.

_____ 1. Exercise can help your skeletal structure (bones).
_____ 2. There are seven basic food groups.
_____ 3. Exercise can help your heart work more effectively.
_____ 4. A baked potato is a good source of protein.
_____ 5. The best exercise is the hardest.
_____ 6. Sweets are classified as fats.
_____ 7. Exercise raises your blood cholesterol level.
_____ 8. Too much sugar can cause weight gain.
_____ 9. Exercise temporarily raises your blood pressure.
_____ 10. The food group from which you should eat the most is meat, chicken, and fish.
_____ 11. Some exercises are better than others for building muscles.
_____ 12. You should try to eat no fats to stay healthy.
_____ 13. Cycling is an example of an aerobic exercise.
_____ 14. MyPlace tells you how much cholesterol a food contains.
_____ 15. Flexibility is the ability to move the parts of your body through a full range of motion.

NUTRITION AND EXERCISE ASSESSMENT (CONT.)

MATCHING

Draw a line from the numbered phrase on the left to the letter on the right.

1. Calcium
2. Vitamin A
3. Cholesterol
4. Fats
5. Starches

a. are complex carbohydrates
b. can cause heart disease
c. are okay to eat in small amounts
d. builds strong bones and teeth
e. is found in yellow and orange fruits and vegetables

6. Breads, pasta, cereals, rice
7. Nutrients
8. Fructose, sucrose, glucose
9. Sodium
10. Water

a. are types of sugars
b. we should drink five to eight glasses per day
c. are the largest group on MyPlace
d. are used by the body for energy, growth, and repair
e. is found in table salt

11. Stretching exercises
12. Aerobic exercise
13. Types of physical fitness
14. Ballistic and stationary
15. Body composition

a. sports- and health-related
b. is the percentage of body fat and muscle
c. isometric and isotonic
d. jumping rope
e. build flexibility

ARISE Basic Health 101: Nutrition and Exercise

Quiz and Assessment Answers

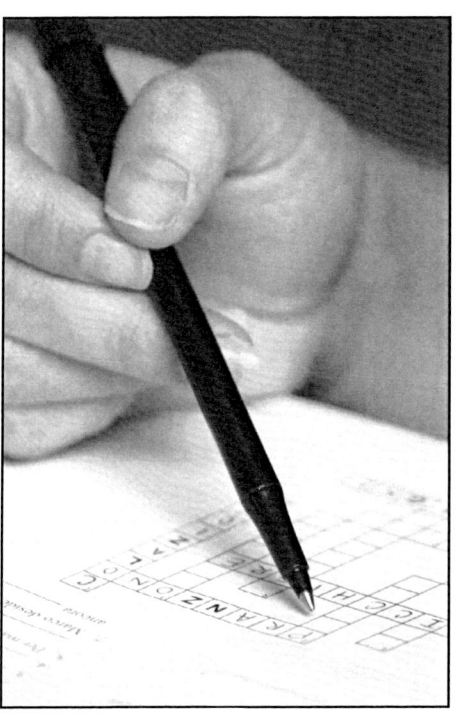

www.ariselife-skills.org

NUTRITION AND EXERCISE ASSESSMENT ANSWERS

True or False:

1. T
2. F
3. T
4. F
5. F
6. T
7. F
8. T
9. T
10. F
11. T
12. F
13. T
14. F
15. T

Matching:

1. D
2. E
3. B
4. C
5. A
6. C
7. D
8. A
9. E
10. B
11. E
12. D
13. A
14. C
15. B

NUTRITION AND EXERCISE QUIZ ANSWERS

Section 1	Section 2	Section 3
1. B	1. A	1. B
2. D	2. B	2. B
3. D	3. C	3. C
4. D	4. A	4. A
5. D	5. B	5. D

DISCUSSION QUESTIONS AND ACTIVITY IDEAS FOR THE ARISE INSPIRATIONAL BIOGRAPHIES

Please Note. If a learner is unable to read or has difficulty reading, make every effort not to embarrass that person. We created these tales specifically for people that have trouble reading and writing. **Do Not Force someone to read who is uncomfortable doing so.**

TECHNIQUES FOR READING THE BIOGRAPHIES

1. The instructor can read the biography out loud.
2. The instructor can call on a volunteer to read the biography.
3. "Jump read" the biography: Have one person begin the story and stop at the end of a thought. Another person jumps in and reads the next thought. This is done until you complete the biography.
4. Have all the learners silently read the biography.
5. Read one paragraph or thought at a time and then ask questions about that thought.

DISCUSSION QUESTIONS

1. What did you learn about the person?
2. What advice do you think the person would give you?
3. What do you remember most about the person after reading his or her biography?
4. What is the person's most significant accomplishment?
5. Would you choose this person to be your friend? Why?

ACTIVITY IDEAS

1. Pretend it is the future. Write your own biography. Be as creative as you want. Here are some questions to get you started:

   - Where do you want to live?
   - What do you want to do for a living?
   - What do you think the world will look like in 20 years? 50 years?
   - Do you see yourself having kids? How many?
   - What will your kids tell people about you?
   - What will your biggest accomplishment be?

2. Create a vision board of what you want your life to look like in the future. Use a large piece of drawing paper. Think about the following and include it on your vision board: Where do you want to live? What type of house do you want? What job do you want? What family do you want around you? How much money do you want to have? What kind of car do you want to drive? Look at the vision board every day as if you already have these things. This helps you focus on what you want rather than what you don't want. (Vision Board activity page immediately follows the biographies.)

ARISE INSPIRATIONAL BIOGRAPHY: JACK LALANNE

"Godfather of Fitness" Jack LaLanne was born in San Francisco on September 26, 1914. When he was a child, LaLanne suffered fits of rage and wild mood swings. At 15, he went to hear a nutritionist speak about sugar addiction. LaLanne figured out that he was eating too much sugar and decided to remake himself into an example of health and fitness.

This was back in the 1930s, when bodybuilding, fitness and proper nutrition were not talked about at all. LaLanne helped design many of the weightlifting machines now found in gyms all over the world. When he was only 21 years old, LaLanne opened the first modern health club in the United States.

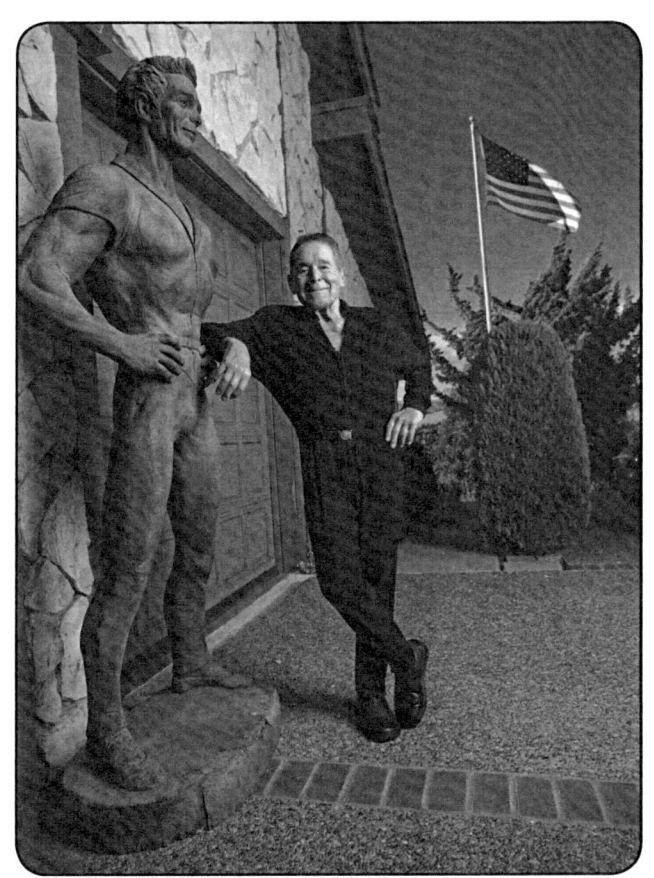

In 1951, LaLanne became the first television fitness instructor. The show ran for 34 years. It allowed LaLanne to branch out into all manner of fitness products, including videos and books.

LaLanne is known for his amazing feats of physical strength. In 1955, he swam from Alcatraz Island to Fisherman's Wharf in San Francisco—while handcuffed. The following year, he performed 1,033 push-ups in 23 minutes on live television, setting a world record.

In 2002, at the age of 88, LaLanne received a star on the Hollywood Walk of Fame. He still works out for two hours every day. Once thought of as odd, LaLanne was far ahead of his time.

"It is most gratifying to me to see that everything I was advocating over 50 years ago, not only exercise-wise but nutrition-wise, is coming to fruition. Back then I was a crackpot. Today, I am an authority. And believe me, I can't die—it would ruin my image!"

ARISE INSPIRATIONAL BIOGRAPHY: VENUS AND SERENA WILLIAMS

Tennis superstars Venus and Serena Williams were born a year apart in the early 1980s. Raised in the crime-ridden Los Angeles suburb of Compton, their father taught them how to play tennis as a way for them to escape their rough neighborhood and have a better life.

The Williams family eventually moved to Florida, and the siblings' tennis careers took off. The pair competed in all the major tennis matches, including the U.S. Open and Wimbledon. The sisters often faced off against each other. In 2002 and 2003, they played each other in four back-to-back Grand Slam Finals—the first siblings to do so. Serena won all four matches. In 2000, the sisters won an Olympic gold medal in women's doubles. Venus was the first African-American to reach the number one ranking in either the men's or women's game. Serena has won more prize money since she started playing tennis than any other female athlete. Although they show fierce competitive spirit on the court, off the court, they are close friends.

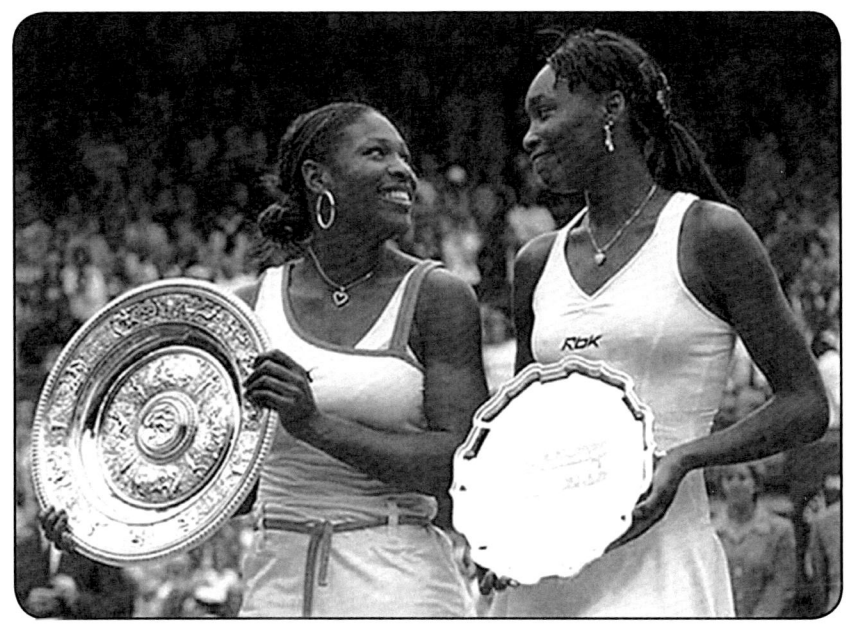

The sisters are also successful businesswomen outside the world of tennis. In 1999, both attended the Art Institute of Florida, where they studied fashion design. Venus runs her own interior design company, called V Starr Interiors, and Serena launched her own clothing line called Aneres. Although a string of injuries in 2006 slowed Venus down, the sisters still live in South Florida and compete all over the world.

ARISE INSPIRATIONAL BIOGRAPHY: JOHN MACKEY AND WHOLE FOODS MARKET

In 1978, 25-year-old college dropout John Mackey and his then-girlfriend borrowed money from family to open up a natural foods store called "SaferWay" in Austin, Texas. The couple were kicked out of their apartment for storing food there, and decided to live in the store. They had to bathe in the store's dishwasher, which had an attached hose.

Two years later, the couple took on two more partners and started the first Whole Foods Market on September 20, 1980. Less than a year later, the store, which had no insurance, was wiped out in a flood. With help from friends, family and volunteers, the store managed to re-open less than a month after the flood.

The Whole Foods mission was to sell food and products that were organic, meaning made with no pesticides or harmful chemicals. Mackey and his partners wanted to create stores that made shopping a fun experience.

"Shopping for groceries for most people is like a chore," Mackey said. "We work at making shopping engaging, fun and interactive."

All the food at Whole Foods has no artificial preservatives, colors or sweeteners. The organic approach is better for the environment. Traditional farming uses chemicals to kill bugs before they destroy the plants. Organic farming uses natural methods to repel pests, eliminating harmful chemical runoff into rivers and oceans.

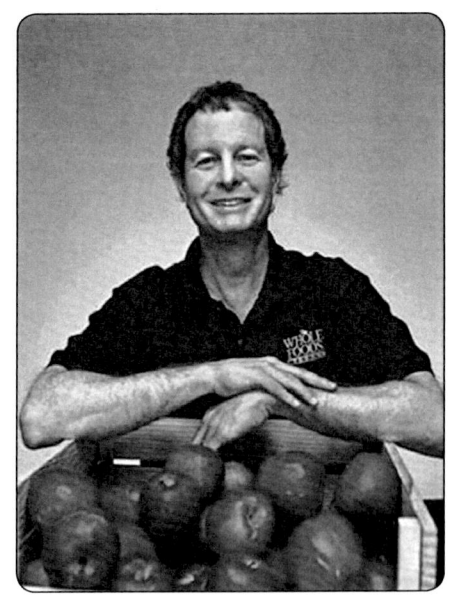

Mackey, who was once criticized for being unrealistic, is now the head of a Fortune 500 company. When he was a kid, he was cut from the school basketball team. He convinced his parents to send him to another school so he could play. That kind of determination is what made him, and Whole Foods Market, such a success.

CREATE YOUR OWN VISION BOARD

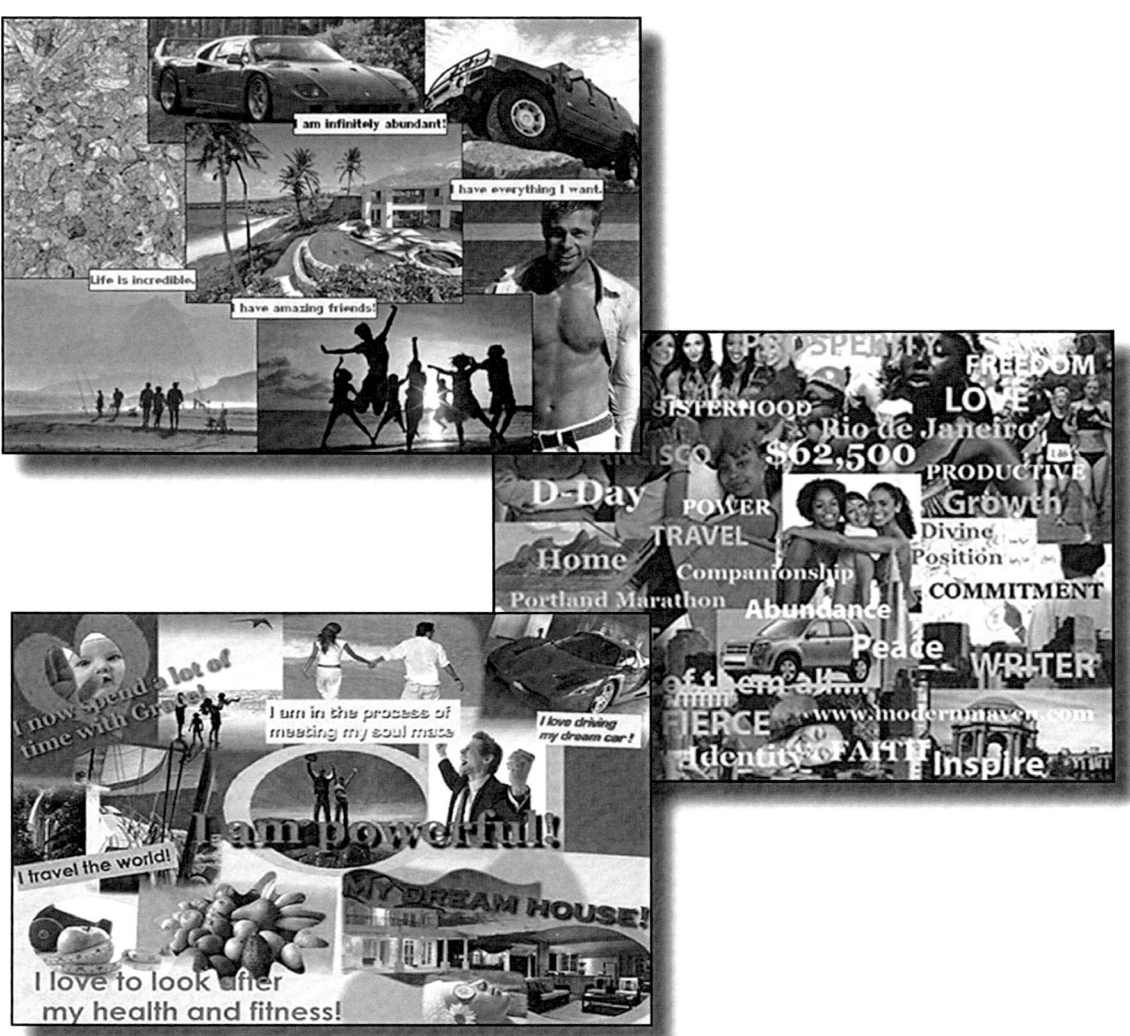

Write down the things you want to include on your vision board, then get started creating it. You can draw pictures, cut out pictures from magazines or take photographs. This is your board to help you visualize your future. See page 115 for more instructions.

_____

_____

_____

USING ARISE TRUE LIFE TALES TO CREATE MEMORABLE LEARNING EXPERIENCES

Please Note. If a learner is unable to read or has difficulty reading, make every effort not to embarrass that person. We created these tales specifically for people that have trouble with reading and writing. **Do Not Force someone to read who is uncomfortable doing so.**

TECHNIQUES FOR READING THE TRUE LIFE TALES

1. The instructor can read the story out loud.
2. The instructor can call on a volunteer to read the story.
3. "Jump read" the story: Have one person begin the story and stop at the end of a thought. Another person jumps in and reads the next thought. This is done until you complete the story.
4. Have all the learners silently read the story.
5. Read one paragraph or thought at a time and then ask questions about that thought.

ACTIVITIES TO DO AFTER THE TRUE LIFE TALES HAVE BEEN READ

1. Group discussion
   a. Ask basic questions relating to who, what, when, where, how, why.
   b. Ask more in-depth questions: What is the difference (between being positive and negative, between staying in school and dropping out?). Use the story: Can you think of a way to handle the situation differently? Explore possibilities: What would have happened if?
2. Create a mind map. A mind map is a diagram used to represent words, ideas and tasks. It is arranged around a central keyword or idea (see example on page 129).
3. Write the following statement on the board and have learners answer it: "This story tells me_____. I can use it in my life to _____."
4. Have the group write a letter to the main character in the story. Tell the character why their story was interesting and decide what the group would have done if they were in the same situation.
5. Create a comic based on the events of the story (see example on page 130).
6. Stop in the middle of the story. Make a prediction as to what you think is going to happen.
7. Have learners create their own "true life tale" to present/act out at their next ARISE group session.
8. Act it out. Create a skit based on the story. First, decide how many characters there are in the story. Assign parts. Skits should not contain violence or inappropriate language or actions. Provide a time limit for preparation and presentation of the skit. Be sure to put quiet people with outgoing people. When performing the skit, learners should use clear voices and the audience should be POLITE.

GREAT OPPORTUNITIES TO USE THE ARISE TRUE LIFE TALES

1. Before the ARISE lesson as a way to grab the learners' attention.
2. In the middle of a lesson as a way to take a small, fun break.
3. As a way to reward people for participation in the ARISE group.
4. As another alternative to engage a quiet group and get people talking.
5. As a way to end a lesson.
6. As a way to give learners experience speaking in front of a group (great for interviewing skills).

26 Bones

My foot is killing me. I mean—it really hurts! I'm stuck in bed. I'm sick of TV and I've read every book and magazine I have. I'm so BORED.

All this could have been avoided, you know.

It happened three days ago.

I stayed up really late playing video games. I was almost at the end of this really hard level, and I just wanted to beat it. Before I knew it, it was three and I was still wide awake. I must have had five or six Cokes that night. All the caffeine kept me awake. I finally fell asleep at five.

At seven, my alarm went off.

Oh, boy, I thought. This was NOT going to be a very good day.

I couldn't stop yawning as I dragged myself around the house, slowly getting ready. I ate a few donuts for breakfast and got in my truck to go to work.

I stopped at the gas station and went inside. I stared at all the energy drinks in the freezer. I usually didn't drink them, because they made my heart race and my hands shake. But this was an emergency. I was too tired to make it through the day. I bought one called "BOLT!"

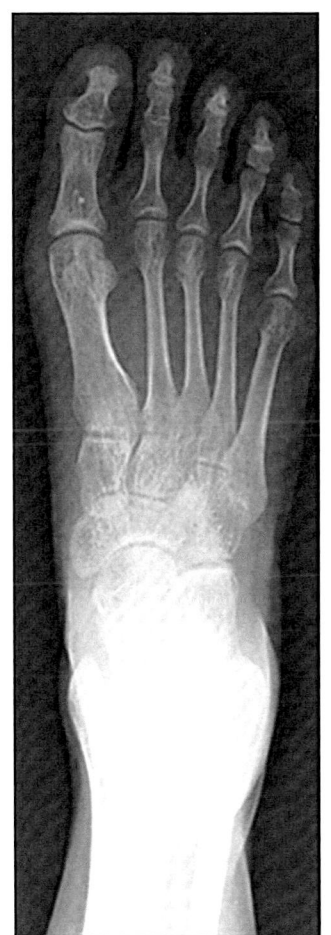

It tasted OK. I drank it down fast as I pulled up to the construction site. My boss was looking at the blueprints. We were building a big parking garage. I waved at him as I punched in and went up to the top floor.

The first two hours were fine. I had plenty of energy. I hammered nails and poured concrete. About three hours into my shift, I started to feel sick. I started to sweat and my arms got a little weak.

Then it happened.

I was carrying a very heavy bag of concrete over to the mixer. I usually use the cart to take the bags over, but I thought I could handle it. If I had slept a normal eight hours the night before, I would have probably been OK. If I wasn't shaky from the energy drink, I could've carried it.

Halfway across the roof of the garage, I dropped the 50-pound bag on my foot.

Pain exploded. I felt the bones break. Do you know how many bones there are in your foot? There are 26.

I broke 24 of them.

Now I'm laying here in the hospital. I broke so many bones that they had to call in a special foot surgeon to fix me.

The worst part is that it's going to cost me a lot to be in the hospital. Since I wasn't using the cart like I was supposed to and I had so much caffeine in my body, my company won't pay for the medical bills.

Plus, I can't work for three months.

If I could go back in time, I would not have played video games all night. I would have gone to bed and slept a good seven hours. I would have eaten a solid breakfast and not been too shaky to work. I definitely would not have bought that crazy energy drink.

That little eight-ounce energy drink ended up costing me thousands of dollars.

I have lots of time to play that video game now—but all I want to do is go back to work.

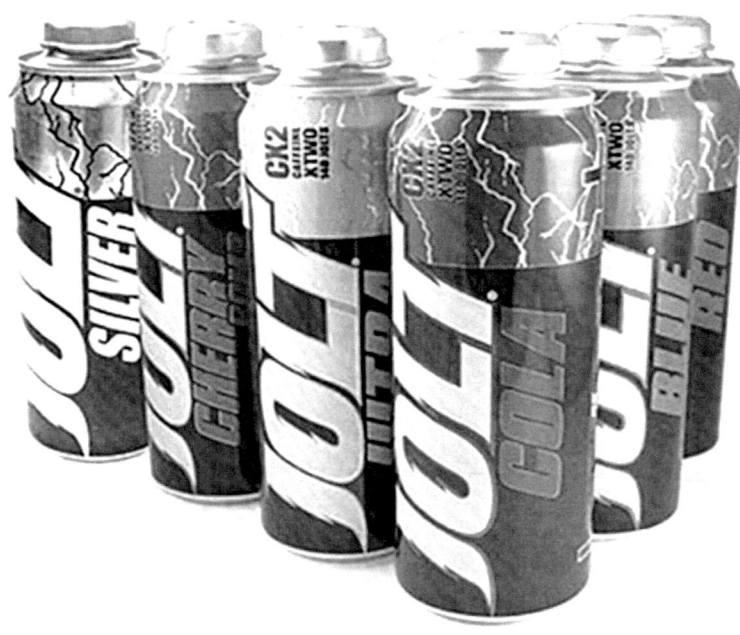

DANCE

I wonder how she did it.

She used to be like me: a little overweight. Tired all the time. Falling asleep in class. She used to sit with us at lunch and feast on cheeseburgers and oily fries and milkshakes. The usual high school lunch junk. We would make excuses to get out of P.E. class. That was last year.

School just started again, and Sara came back in great shape. She is long and thin. Her legs and arms are toned. She must have a workout secret. Maybe she went to the gym everyday. What a crappy way to spend your whole summer! I hate going to the gym. In fact, I don't really like working out at all. I hate boring walks on a treadmill or lifting weights. If you ask me, sweat is the enemy!

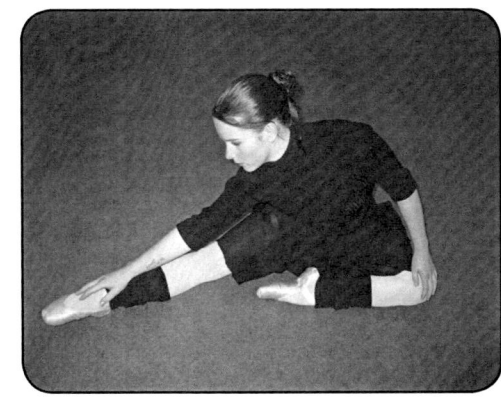

"Hey, Nina!" Sara came up to me today during lunch. She was wearing a skirt that showed off her amazing legs. She was eating a turkey sandwich. I sighed and ate another French fry.

"Hi, Sara."

"I was thinking…want to work out with me after school today?" Sara asked.

She said the "W" word. Ugh. Can't we just eat Oreos and watch Oprah?

"I guess, sure," I said.

"Great. We'll walk to my house after school!"

She bounced off and I glared at my slice of pizza. Great. A math test AND exercise in one day.

After school, we went to Sara's house as planned.

I followed her into the living room. She went over to the stereo and put on a CD.

Let the torture begin!

The music started. It had a great beat and I felt my foot tapping on its own.

Sara started to move. She began to dance. Slow at first, but as the music got faster, so did she. She closed her eyes and was in her own world, moving and shaking to the beat. I couldn't help but start to dance too. The music was too good to ignore. I started to sweat as I moved all over the room.

We danced through five songs. Sweat poured down my back, but I felt great. It didn't feel like exercise at all. It just felt like getting into the music and letting it carry you away.

"See?" she said with a huge smile as she shut off the CD player and handed me a glass of water. "Exercise doesn't have to be boring. You don't even have to go to the gym to get a good workout."

"No?"

"Nope," she said, smiling. "All you have to do is dance."

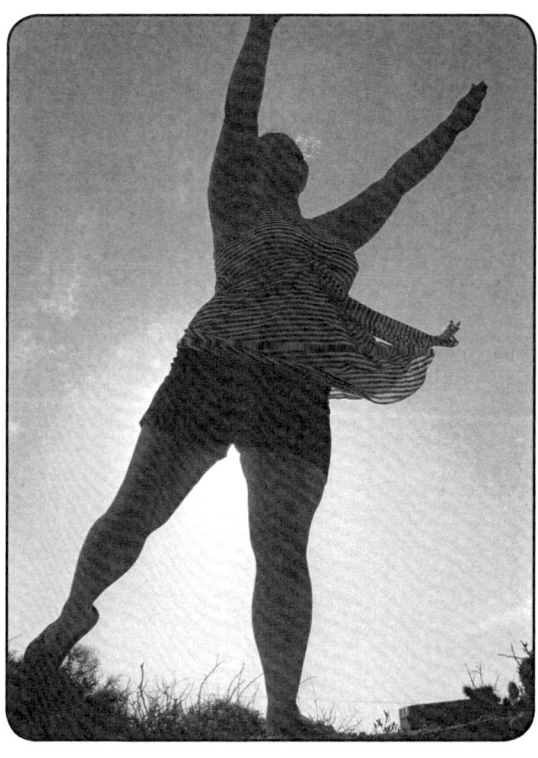

NEEDLES

I really hate needles.

You do too?

Then you better take care of yourself! You might end up like me, having to face down a needle every single day.

Let me tell you a little story. When I was growing up, my family was overweight. We ate fried chicken, sugary breakfast cereals, bacon and all sorts of other fatty foods. Before I knew it, I was the "chubby kid" at school. The boys made fun of me and the girls ignored me. So, I would come home and cry while I ate leftover pizza and bags of potato chips.

I grew into a very fat woman. By the time I graduated high school, I weighed well into my 300's. I had to buy clothes from a special store. People stared at me. My knees and back ached all the time. I would get winded walking from my car into the grocery store. And stairs? Forget it.

Worst of all—I felt bad. I was always tired. I felt totally worthless.

Well, one day I went to the doctor. I had been feeling completely exhausted. I was always thirsty and had to use the restroom constantly. My vision was a little blurry. It was starting to scare me, so I made an appointment. I had not been to a doctor in over five years.

Dr. Maddow welcomed me into his office. He listened as I told him my symptoms. He ran some blood work. A few days later, he asked me to come back.

"Melina," he said, "You have type 2 diabetes. Do you know what that is?"

"No," I said. But I knew it wasn't good.

"Type 2 diabetes is a disease that causes your body to have trouble digesting sugar. In your case, extra body fat has caused your pancreas to stop making insulin, or sugar, the way it needs to."

"What do I need to do?" I asked.

"Well, unfortunately, you're going to have to start checking your blood sugar every few hours and giving yourself insulin shots. You must go on a very strict diet. You have to exercise every day."

I started to cry. I had to stick myself with a needle a few times every single day?

The nurses taught me how to inject myself. Man, it hurt. They gave me insulin, needles, an insulin meter and pamphlets on diet and exercise.

For someone who hated needles, having type 2 diabetes was very hard. My blood sugar was always low, so I had to inject myself three times a day. It never got easier. The needles always hurt.

I resolved to get healthy. Dr. Maddow told me that if I didn't start eating right and exercising, I would die. How's that for motivation?

The first six months after I was told I had diabetes, I lost almost 100 pounds. I worked hard.

Know what my motivation was? Those needles!

I walked every day. I started out just walking to the end of the driveway and back. Now I'm up to almost four miles a day. I dumped all the fast food, sugar, white flour and red meat from my diet. Carrot sticks are my friends now! Can you believe it?

As my weight dropped, so did my need for insulin injections. Dr. Maddow says that if I lose another 30 pounds, I might be able to manage my diabetes with diet and exercise alone.

Hopefully, I'll be able to stop the injections soon. I hope you learn from my story, so needles don't become part of your everyday life. Trust me, it's MUCH easier to eat healthy and exercise than to deal with diabetes.

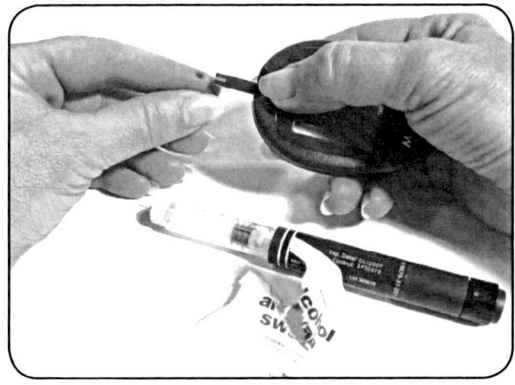

SMILE

Ever have trouble sleeping?

I sure used to.

I would lie in bed all night, unable to turn off my thoughts, staring at the ceiling. I watched the minutes click by on the digital clock. They were like little red eyes staring at me in the dark, wondering why I was still awake when the rest of the world was sleeping.

I tried everything I could think of: warm milk, hot baths, drops of lavender on my pillow, counting sheep. None of it worked. I could have tried sleeping pills, but I didn't want to risk getting addicted. Eventually I gave up and started filling my nights with online video games and infomercials.

I went through my days in a fog. I lived on a constant caffeine buzz. My hands shook and my heart pounded in my chest. If I cut out caffeine, I started to drag and got wicked headaches.

After two months of losing sleep, I decided to take a vacation. I went to visit my grandfather at the Navajo reservation in New Mexico. He took one look at me and knew something was terribly wrong.

"Why do you look so worn out?" he said in his deep, baritone voice. I looked up at him. His face was leathery and kind. His eyes were the darkest blue, just like mine.

"Thoughts get in my head and I can't get them out," I said. "They just run around and around in there, like a hamster on a wheel. Before I know it, the whole night has passed and I'm still awake."

"Thomas," he said, "You need to smile."

"Grandpa, I don't think smiling would help."

"Yes, it will," he argued. "What you do is you lie in bed. Whenever an unwelcome thought comes into your mind, you smile. A smile tricks your mind into forgetting whatever you were just thinking. Your mind wants to match a thought to that smile. So you stop thinking negative things and you suddenly think good, smiling thoughts. You breathe, focusing on each breath going in and out and imagining the energy moving down through your hands and feet. And you smile."

"Oh, come on, Gramps," I sighed. "It can't be that easy."

"Try it tonight," he said. He left to feed his horses.

That night, I lay in bed staring at the ceiling, as usual. I thought about everything that scared me: global warming, the economy, dating, high cholesterol, new brakes for my car…everything.

I sat up and forced myself to smile.

My mind went totally blank. I smiled and smiled. While that smile was on my face, I couldn't seem to come up with a negative thought. Instead, my brain was calm. The scattered thoughts dissolved. It felt strange to keep smiling, but I made myself do it. My breath slowed and I began to relax.

My eyelids grew heavy. I laid my head down on the pillow and a warm rush of relief filled me as I drifted off to sleep. At last.

The next morning, I came out of the bedroom bright-eyed and cheerful.

"You smiled your way to sleep, didn't you?" Grandfather asked, flipping corncakes on the stove.

I nodded.

"It works anytime, you know," he said. "If you are feeling overwhelmed or stressed, just smile until you forget why you felt that way. How do you think I've lived so long?"

I didn't have an answer for that. I could only smile.

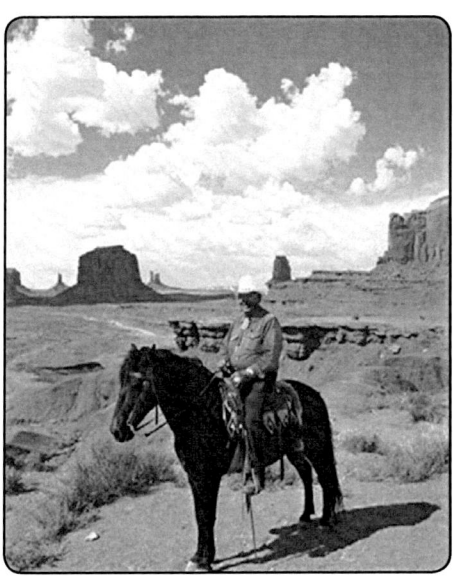

CREATE A MIND MAP

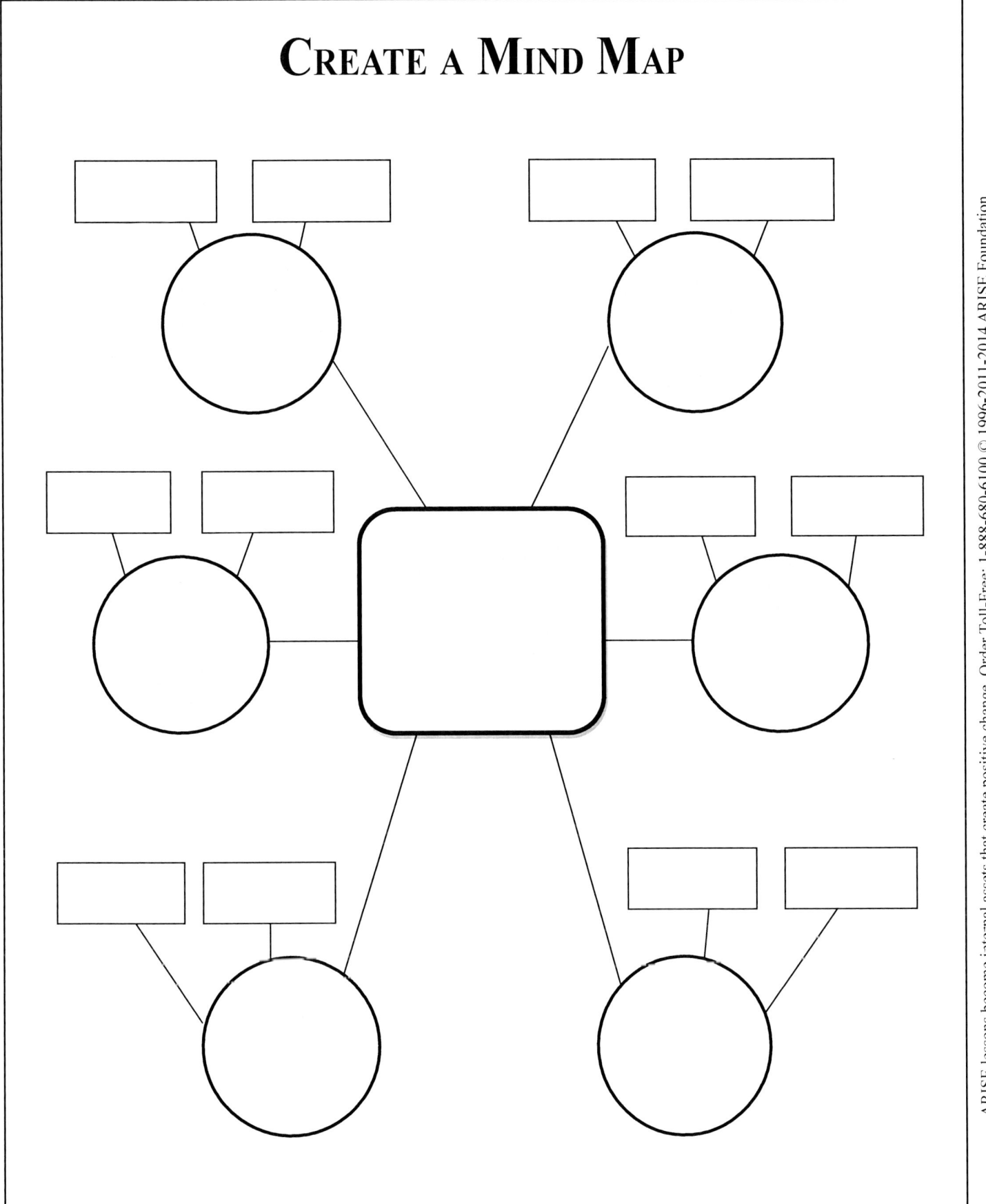

ARISE Basic Health 101: Nutrition and Exercise, Instructor's Manual, Page 129

DRAW A COMIC

Based on the story you just read. Not everyone is an artist. Do the best you can.

How to Make The Most of the ARISE Life Quotes Found Throughout this Manual

You will find ARISE Life Quotes throughout this manual. Quotes can be used to enhance the lesson idea. A quote, or quotation, is a piece of writing that helps explain a point. It also introduces learners to well-known people from history or modern life. The learners can find out about the person being quoted. It can enhance their knowledge of the world around them.

ARISE Life Quotes are wonderful little things:
- They can convey a world of meaning in just a few words.
- Quotes provide inspiration and guidance.
- Quotes can motivate learners, like recharging a battery.
- Quotes can be found everywhere: books, greeting cards, websites and daily emails, just to name a few.

How to use the ARISE Life Quotes:
1. Have a group discussion on the meaning of the quote. This can be done as a whole group, in small groups or in pairs.
2. Ask learners to read the quote, then write the meaning of the quote in their own words.
3. Instruct learners to illustrate the quote on a large piece of paper using their own colors and lettering. They can draw pictures around the quote to make it into a piece of art.
4. Learners can practice dramatically reading the quote, and then have volunteers present their "performance" to the group.
5. Encourage each learner to create and decorate a quote folder. They can collect quotes that are important to them and keep them to refer to.
6. Use a quote to introduce and highlight an activity. This can help make a lesson even more memorable. A quote can also sum up the lesson.
7. Ask your learners to get a small notebook. Every time a quote comes into their lives, encourage them to write it in their quote books. Whenever they need inspiration, they can read their quote book.
8. When you have a small window of time, like after a lesson break, fill it with a quote.
9. Discuss learners' favorite quotes.

Where to find additional Quotes:
- Type "Quotes," "Famous Quotes," "Inspirational Quotes" or "Quotes on (a specific topic)" into Google, Yahoo search, AOL search, etc.
- Libraries and bookstores are stocked with books on quotations. They are usually found in the reference section. Ask a staff member for help.
- Newspapers and magazines might have quotes.

For more useful quotes, please order ARISE Get Smart! Series, Volume 6, "ARISE Secrets of Success Quotes" on the ARISE website: http://www.ariselife-skills.org

HOW TO EFFECTIVELY USE THE ARISE MOTIVATIONAL POSTERS IN THIS MANUAL

You will find many useful ARISE posters throughout this manual. The posters can be used to create a lesson or they can provide an interesting visual aid to enhance the subject area you are teaching.

ARISE posters offer a quick lesson:

- They visually present something you want learners to learn quickly.
- They provide information to use when making choices.
- Posters can motivate quickly just by looking at them.
- You can find many additional posters on our website: www.ariselife-skills.org.

How to use the ARISE posters:

1. Develop a series of questions related to the poster:

   - Ask questions that require a yes or no answer first, as they are nonthreatening. The youth can answer without too much personal risk.
   - Ask who, what, when, where, how and why questions.
   - Ask questions that probe (Do you think...?; What do you assume from this poster?).
   - Ask questions about personal meaning (What does this poster mean to you?).
   - Ask questions that show consequences (What would happen if you did …?).

2. Have the learners create their own poster on the same topic.

3. Have the learners create a rap on the topic of the poster.

4. Brainstorm. Write the title of the poster on the board or large piece of paper. Have the learners tell you all they know about the topic of the poster and write their answers on the chart. Each of their answers can become a discussion topic. Create a mind map as a form of brainstorming.

5. Divide your learners into groups and have each group come up with a one-sentence summary of the meaning of the poster. A one-sentence summary is: This poster tells me_____ and I can use it in my life to _____.

6. Have the learners create a skit that tells the meaning of the poster.

For additional motivational posters, visit the ARISE website: www.ariselife-skills.org

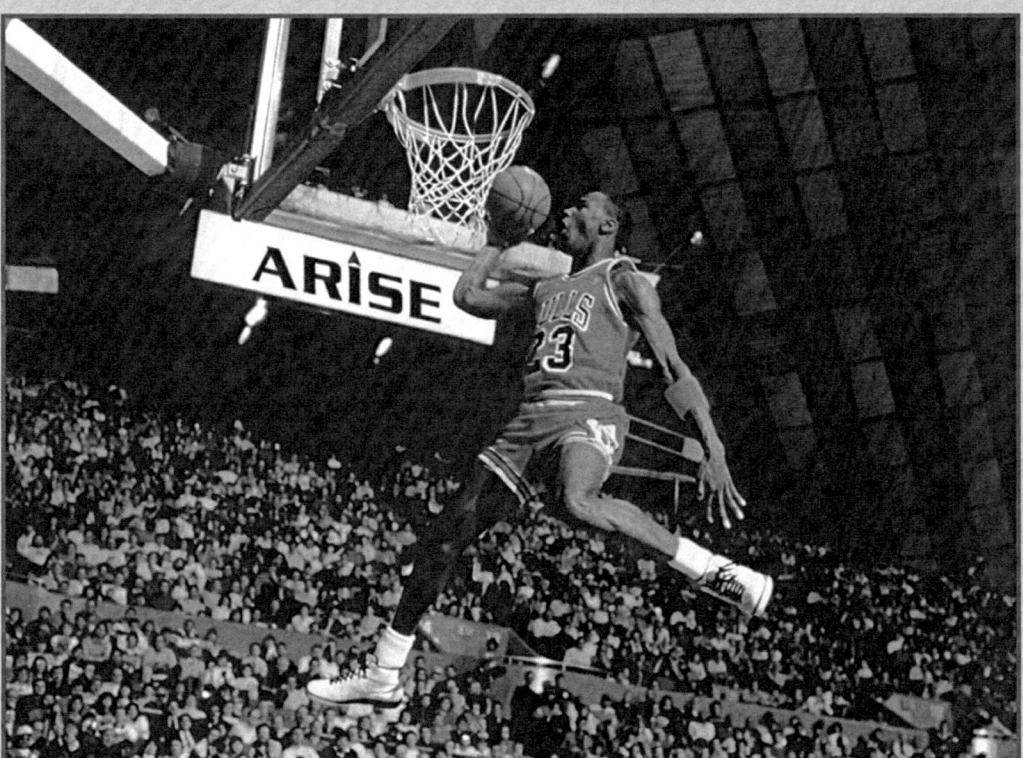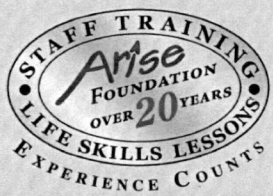

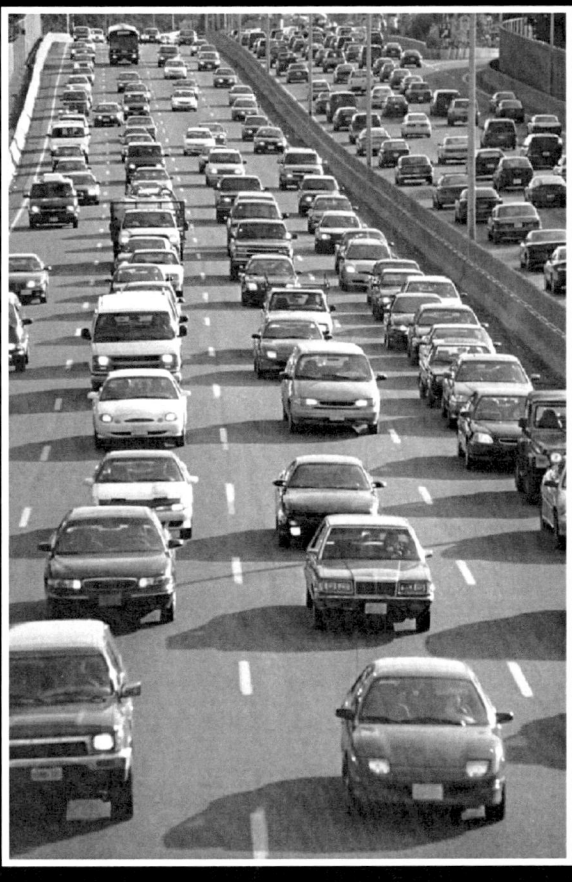
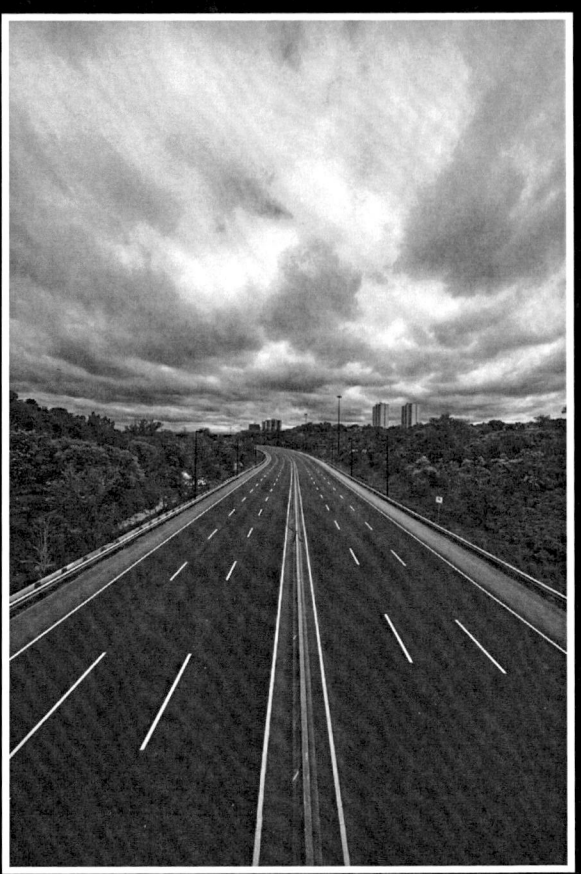

EXERCISE CAN REVERSE CLOGGED ARTERIES

FOOD IS FUEL

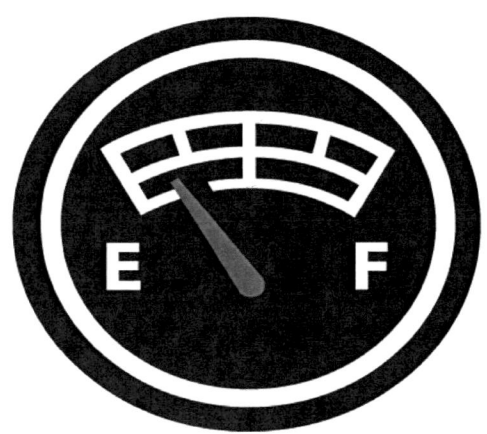

ARE YOU RUNNING ON EMPTY CALORIES?

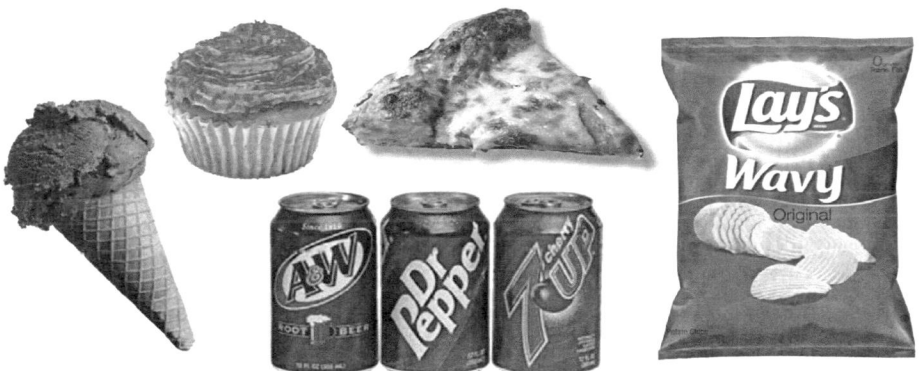

Order Toll Free 1-888-680-6100   www.ariselife-skills.org

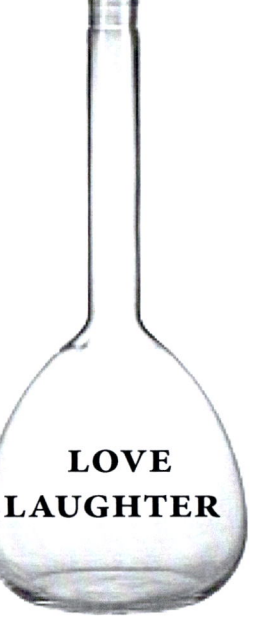

ARISE TEEN CURRICULA

ARISE Work in Progress:
- Book 1: Anger Management
- Book 2: Substance Abuse and Guns
- Book 3: Domestic & Sexual Abuse
- Book 4: Violence & Conflict

ARISE Four-Wheel Drive For the Mind
- Book 1: Self Esteem
- Book 2: Learning Strategies & Time Management
- Book 3: Networking, Jobs & Money

ARISE Basic Health 101
- Book 1: Health & Hygiene
- Book 2: Nutrition & Exercise

ARISE Official Homo Sapiens Operator's Manual
- Book 1: Parts & Operations
- Book 2: Maintaining Your Homo Sapiens Equipment
- Book 3: Take The Highway to Health
- Book 4: Official Homo Sapiens Family Medical Records
- Official Homo Sapiens Vocabulary Book

ARISE So You're Thinking of Dropping Out of School? (Dropping Out Vol. I)

ARISE So You're Thinking of Staying in School? (Dropping Out Vol. II)

ARISE Brainfood
- Book 1: Peaceful Living
- Book 2: Creating a Positive Outlook
- Book 3: Supercharging Your System
- Book 4: Being Safe
- Book 5: More Secrets of Success
- Book 6: The Right Stuff & Money Matters

ARISE Sprouts: A Teen Pregnancy Prevention Program
- Book 1: Prenatal, Delivery, Postpartum and Mental Development
- Book 2: Physical and Emotional Development
- Book 3: Building a Family & Teen Pregnancy
- Book 4: Child Safety
- Book 5: Are You Living an Upside-Down Life?

ARISE Fatherhood
ARISE Domestic Abuse
ARISE Rules of the Road

ARISE TEEN CURRICULA

10-20-Life
Only Joking? There's Nothing Funny About Threats
31 of Taneka's Urban Life Tales
Gangs: 50 + Stories of Fractured Lives
ARISE Teen Anger Danger
Life Isn't Fair

ARISE Get Smart! Series 1-6
Tips for Teaching ARISE Get Smart!

VIDEOS:
- Anger Management & Meditation Video
- ARISE Basic STD Class Video
- Friendly Foods Video
- Smart Car Shopping Video
- Stay in School Video
- Why Spend Your Life in a Cage? Video

OTHER ARISE Items:
- ARISE Training Manual & DVD
- Tips for Teaching ARISE Videos
- ARISE Motivational Posters in the following sizes:
    - 11" X 17"
    - 12" X 18"
    - 24" X 36"

ARISE MIDDLE SCHOOL CURRICULA

ARISE Life Skills for Middle School Volumes 1-4
ARISE When There's Trouble, Who Do You Call?

ARISE Rescue Me: Mother Earth Dials 911
Book 1: The Environmental Basics
Book 2: What's Hurting Me

ARISE On Stage
ARISE Life Isn't Fair
ARISE Living a Healthy Lifestyle

ARISE PRE-K - 5th GRADE CURRICULA

ARISE Little by Little: Pre-K
- Book 1: Me and My Emotions
- Book 2: My Character and Ethics
- Book 3: Me and My World
- Book 4: Keeping Me Safe
- Book 5: A Healthy Me

ARISE Little by Little K - Grade 1
- Book 1: Safety All Around
- Book 2: My Character and Ethics
- Book 3: All About Me
- Art Activity Book and Puppet Plays Book

ARISE Life Skills for Young Folks, Grades 2 - 3 (Vol. 1 - 2)

ARISE Big Kids Book of Life's Lessons, Grades 4 - 5 (Vol. 1 - 2)

ARISE Child Safety Event Weeks, Grades 3 - 5

Auto Safety	Anti-graffiti
Burn Awareness	Electrical Safety
Stranger Safety	Gun Awareness
Health Awareness	Poison Prevention
Substance Abuse Awareness	Lead Awareness
Violence Reduction and Anger Management	Success

Kid's Alert
The Big ARISE Safety Book
ABC Word Games
Stranger Safety Coloring Book
The Write Stuff

ARISE Videos for Pre-K through 5th Grade

Graffiti No!
No to Guns!
Drugs, No Way!
Stranger Safety
Safe, Snug and Secure
Where the Waste Goes
Poison Look-a-Likes

OTHER ARISE Items:

ARISE Songs for Making Good Choices
ARISE Sing-Along CD
ARISE Motivational Posters

ARISE Life Skills Facilitator Training

The ARISE Life-Skills Training certifies participants as ARISE Life-Skills Group Facilitators (ALSGFs). It is designed specifically for those who have no formal experience, but who are eager to teach life skills to at-risk youth, particularly those with behavior issues and learning disabilities. The training experience is highly interactive, with many opportunities to practice newfound coaching skills that hold the interest of troubled youth turned off by the usual classroom activities. Learners discover the ease with which the ARISE Formula promotes high levels of positive interaction with youth in group settings.

In addition to learning how to conduct these breakthrough lessons, participants will learn group facilitation skills and non-confrontational methods for handling troubled, disinterested, and disruptive youth. This training is a must for utilizing the ARISE life-skills curriculum to its fullest potential.

Additional benefits include a reduction in staff frustration levels, turnover, and friction with youth in their charge.

Ideal for:

- Juvenile Justice Staff
- Therapists
- Religious Leaders
- Social Service Personnel
- School Counselors
- Teachers
- School Resource Officers and Police Officers
- Probation Officers
- Human Resources
- Social Workers
- School Administrators
- Case Managers
- Community-Based Programs
- Youth with Mental Health Issues
- Halfway Houses
- Anyone Interested in Helping At-Risk Youth

The ARISE Life Skills training is available as an **onsite training**: http://at-riskyouth.org/training/arise-2-day-life-skills-group-facilitator-training/ or as an **online training**: http://at-riskyouth.org/arise-e-learning/arise-life-skills-e-training/.

For more information, visit the ARISE website:
www.ariselife-skills.org or call toll-free: 1 (888) 680-6100.

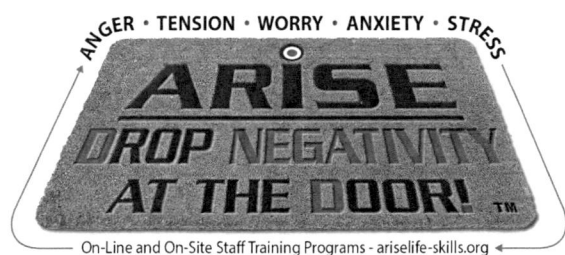

ARISE
Drop It at the Door

An Uncommon Program for Uncommon Times

ARISE Certified Drop It at The Door training provides participants with the tools needed to handle the anger, stress at work, worry, anxiety and guilt awaiting us as we open the doors to work and home.

ARISE Drop It at The Door participants not only hear what is being said, those fortunate enough to participate have their memories stimulated by rich visuals that make a positive and lasting impression.

The ARISE workshop guarantees that participants will leave with a brand new set of tools enabling them to drop negativity at the door, comfortably manage stress at work, guilt, worrying, anxiety and anger in their work and home life relationships.

TOPICS:

- What is anger? (What does it look like, feel like, etc.)
- Why are we getting angry? What's going on in our lives?
- How does anger affect us physically and emotionally?
- What do peace and happiness feel like?
- Techniques for "Dropping It at The Door!"

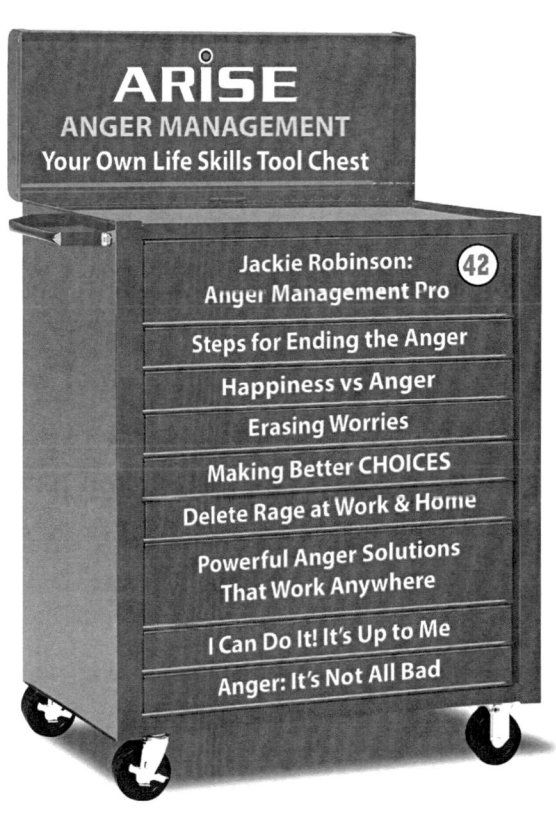

ARISE Basic Health 101: Nutrition and Exercise, Instructor's Manual, Page 141

- Living a happier, more fulfilling life
- Dropping negativity
- Using positive thinking tools and techniques
- Improving personal and professional relationships
- Paying it forward

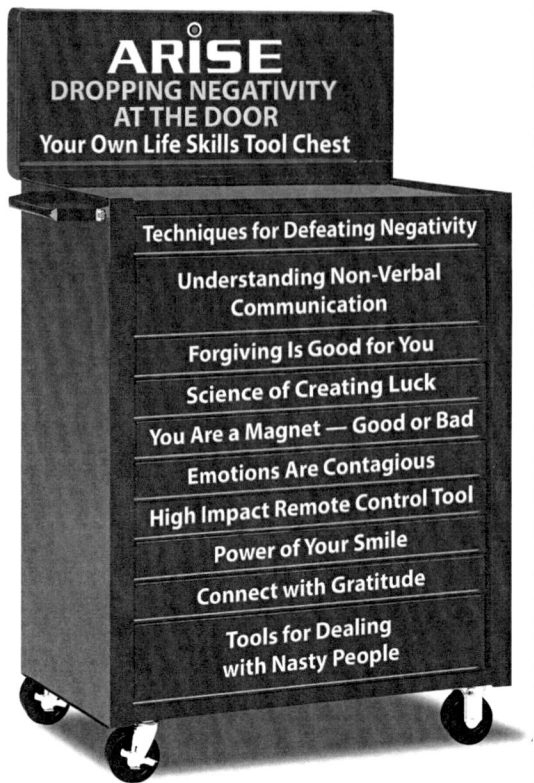

Additional topics can be seen at: http://at-riskyouth.org/training/drop-it-at-the-door/days/.

The ARISE Drop It at The Door training is available as an **onsite training** for 2 days or 5 days: http://at-riskyouth.org/training/drop-it-at-the-door/ or as an **online training**: http://at-riskyouth.org/arise-e-learning/arise-life-skills-e-training/.

For more information, visit the ARISE website: www.ariselife-skills.org or call toll-free: 1 (888) 680-6100.

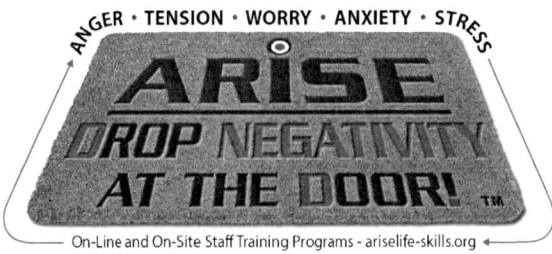